The Thyroid, Cancer and You

The Thyroid, Cancer and You

Knowledge is Power!
How Much Do You Know?

A. Wolfe

To order additional copies of this book, contact:

Xlibris Corporation
1-888-795-4274
www.Xlibris.com
Orders@Xlibris.com
21750

Contents

This book is dedicated to:

My Family,
Who stood by me, and supported me during this very difficult time in all
of our lives.
For their many prayers and thoughtfulness,
for enduring the many hours of research that went into this book,
For welcoming some of the changes in our diet,
and for taste testing the meals to get the recipes
for this book just right!

My Church Family
who diligently supported, prayed for,
and helped with even
the day-to-day needs of our family.

Dr. Marjorie Safran, Dr. Nilima Patwardhan, and
Dr. Kathryn Cohan.
For their dedication to their profession
and to their patients.
Also for their support, encouragement and empathy.

My Lord and Savior Jesus Christ
without whom I could not have come through this,
His mercy is new every morning.
Without Him I could not share this wealth of information
with all of you.

"For I know the plans I have for you,"
declares the Lord,
"plans to prosper you and not to harm you,
plans to give you hope and a future."
Jeremiah 29:11

Greetings

Greetings Fellow Seeker of Knowledge,

Since you are reading this book you have or know someone who has a thyroid disorder and has probably been diagnosed with Thyroid Cancer, or you are a close family member or friend of someone who has. Whether you are any of these, this book is written for YOU. The thyroid gland and its disorders are not widely understood among the general public. I became aware of how little I knew as I began to research this gland that brought about the biggest single change to my physical body and my life.

I want to begin by talking a little bit about the thyroid, what it does and about some of the common disorders. Then I want to talk about thyroid cancer. And last but not least, the things we can do to help our bodies fight diseases such as this cancer.

Included in this book is useful information and discussion followed by a recipe section (with variations) to take you through your "low iodine" diet (which is required for cancer treatment and screening) with **maximum benefits** to your immune system. The variations will help further enhance your immune system beyond the diet.

We've all heard, "If I only knew then what I know now." Well here's your chance. Having gone through the disorders then the cancer and treatment has given me a desire to give you information and discuss with you things that "I wish I'd known then."

Your immune system has to be a priority because that is what you have been given to fight and to conquer disease.

I am a thyroid cancer survivor, who has experienced the heartache of diagnosis, preparations, biopsies, surgery, radiation treatments and follow-up scans. As I said before there is much I would like to share with you.

The multitude of thoughts and questions that immediately come to mind can be nearly overwhelming. It is very hard to think when you get this diagnosis. What exactly does it mean to have Thyroid Cancer? It doesn't mean what it used to but it is still very, very serious. I would like to share with you things I wish had been shared with me. There is so much the experience has taught me during the time of trying to diagnose the problem, the possible diagnosis of cancer, the preparation for the surgery, the surgery itself, the diagnosis and then the radiation treatment, which I was poorly prepared for.

The material contained in this book is intended for informational purposes only. I have no medical training. I am not engaged in rendering medical advice or professional services. This information should **not** be used for diagnosing or treating thyroid cancer! *It is **not** a substitute for professional care.* And before beginning any new diet and/or exercise program, consult your physician.

This book will take you through a journey that is interactive in nature. I want you to take this book with you to the doctor's office. There is a section for you to write down notes and information. It seems that information gets jumbled as you are trying to sort through it all and file it in your mind. It is helpful to have information on hand to carry with you.

There is so much information on the thyroid gland that I cannot cover in this book. Many medical journals have been written on the information in this book. I can only give you an overview and hopefully inspire you to seek more knowledge, not just about the thyroid gland, but knowledge about your own body. Taking responsibility for your health is not an easy road, but it is well worth the effort and has many benefits and rewards. Let's start our search for knowledge with the thyroid gland itself.

The Thyroid

The Thyroid

The thyroid is a butterfly shaped gland that is situated just below your "Adam's Apple" or larynx, normally weighing less than one ounce. It is the biggest gland in the neck. It is made up of two halves, called lobes, which wrap around the windpipe (trachea) and are joined together by a narrow band of thyroid tissue, known as the isthmus. It affects heart rate, cholesterol level, body weight, energy level, muscle strength, skin condition, vision, menstrual regularity, mental state and a host of other conditions.

The thyroid gland is under the control of the pituitary gland, a small gland the size of a peanut at the base of the brain. The pituitary gland is regulated by another gland known as the hypothalamus, which is part of the brain and produces TRH (thyrotropin releasing hormone). When the level of thyroid hormones (T4 & T3) drops too low the hypothalamus sends a signal to the pituitary gland to produce TSH (thyroid stimulating hormone). When the pituitary gland receives the signal it releases TSH to the thyroid gland.

When the thyroid receives TSH, it responds by releasing two of its own hormones, T4 (thyroxine) and T3 (Triiodothyronine), which enter the bloodstream and affect the metabolism of the heart, liver, muscles and other organs. The pituitary gland acts as a monitor of thyroid hormone levels in the blood and increases or decreases the amount of TSH that is released, which then changes the amount of thyroid hormone in the blood. Basically every cell in the body depends on the thyroid hormones for regulation of their metabolism. The normal thyroid gland produces about 80% T4 and about 20% T3. T3, however, possesses about four times the hormone strength of T4.

The function of the thyroid gland is to take iodine, found in many foods, and convert it into the above-mentioned thyroid hormones, T4 and T3. Thyroid cells are the only cells that absorb iodine. The thyroid cells combine the iodine with an amino acid called tyrosine to make the T4 and T3 hormones. I want to repeat that every cell in the body depends on thyroid hormone for the regulation of its metabolism.

TSH testing is very important for the general public, especially the adult population. TSH tests, due to their high degree of sensitivity, allow physicians to diagnose thyroid disorders at an early stage, even before patients begin to experience symptoms. In the past, doctors were unable to diagnose thyroid disorders until a patient showed fairly advanced symptoms.

A Johns Hopkins University study that was published in *the Journal of the American Medical Association* proposes routine testing for mild thyroid failure. Their study concluded that periodic screening of men and women, age thirty-five years and older at regular intervals is as effective a health strategy as screening for more common medical conditions such as high cholesterol or high blood pressure. The study involved the use of the TSH test, to provide the most accurate measure of thyroid gland activity. Since most physicians do not routinely do this test, which is administered by drawing a small blood sample, you should ask for this to be done at your annual physical even if you are not experiencing any signs or symptoms of thyroid disease or thyroid disorders. Most endocrinologists believe that TSH levels rise when a person is in the earliest stages of thyroid failure.

There are many thyroid conditions that I would like to mention before I present the cancer factor. There are thyroid goiters, there are thyroid nodules, there is hypothyroidism (the most common thyroid condition), there is hyperthyroidism there is thyroiditis and others. Then there is thyroid cancer.

Thyroid Disorders

Thyroid Disorders

The thyroid gland contains two main types of cells. *Thyroid follicular cells* make and store thyroid hormone. They also make a special thyroid protein called *thyroglobulin.* *C-Cells* make another hormone called *calcitonin.* Different cancers develop from each type of cell. Their differences determine the seriousness of the cancer and the required treatment. Because the thyroid gland is close to the skin, tumors can appear as bumps in the neck that you can feel. These are called thyroid *nodules*, and can develop at any age. I had one at age sixteen. Thyroid nodules commonly arise on an otherwise normal thyroid gland. They are often located at the edge of the thyroid gland so they can be felt as a lump in the throat. Nodules can be as simple as an overgrowth of normal thyroid tissue.

Almost ninety-five percent of thyroid *nodules* or tumors are benign. *Multinodular goiter* describes a thyroid with several benign *nodules*. Often they are cysts that contain fluid, or they are lumps of stored thyroid hormone called *colloid nodules*. Around five percent of the thyroid nodules are cancerous. Some statistics that I found interesting were that one in twelve to fifteen women has a thyroid nodule. One in forty to fifty men has a thyroid nodule.

More than ninety percent of all thyroid nodules are benign (non-cancerous). Most are actually cysts, which are filled with fluid rather than thyroid tissue. That is the type of nodule I had later, in my early twenties. Usually a fine needle aspiration biopsy will tell if the nodule is cancerous or not. (Other tests include Thyroid scan, Thyroid biopsy, and Thyroid ultrasonography.) Initially I had hyperthyroidism, most likely secondary to the toxic nodule. Radioactive iodine was used to treat the hyperthyroidism. This treatment essentially "shuts down" thyroid hormone production. Normal hormone levels are often restored through levothyroxine sodium tablets. Follow-up all through your lifetime is critical to ensure you are receiving the proper dosage of this thyroid medication. Radioactive iodine therapy is still the treatment of choice in most cases. I had this treatment and would not recommend this to anyone. The radioactive iodine treatment given to me shut down only one half of my thyroid and no thyroid hormone was given. When my cancer was diagnosed I also had cancer in the half of my thyroid that was supposedly "shut down."

A *thyroid goiter* is an enlargement of the thyroid gland, usually dramatic. It is not associated with overproduction of thyroid hormone or malignancy. There are a number of factors, which may cause the thyroid to become enlarged. One is a diet deficient in iodine, but this is rarely the cause because of readily available iodine in our diets. Another cause and more common is an increase in thyroid stimulating hormone (TSH). Something happens within the normal synthesis within the thyroid. The TSH as we mentioned earlier comes from the pituitary gland. This enlargement usually takes years to be seen. There is no limit to how large a goiter can get, so surgical removal is often recommended. This is to relieve the compression of the trachea and esophagus. Small to moderate sized goiters can be treated successfully with thyroid hormone replacement therapy. This is in the form of a pill. By supplying thyroid hormone, the pituitary will make less TSH, which could result in stabilizing the thyroid and will often cause the size of the goiter to decrease.

There are diseases of the thyroid that are not cancerous but are very serious in nature. One of these is hyperthyroidism and of this type the most serious is called ***"Graves' disease"***. This is caused by generalized over activity of the entire thyroid gland. It is also called "diffuse toxic goiter." "Diffuse" because the entire thyroid gland is involved; "toxic" because the patient appears hot and flushed, as if feverish due to an infection; and "goiter" because the thyroid gland enlarges in this condition. In Graves' disease, antibodies are produced against certain proteins on the surface of thyroid cells, stimulating those cells to overproduce thyroid hormones resulting in an overactive thyroid. The exact cause is not understood, but the immune system can produce antibodies that invade and attack the thyroid. Current research validates that this disease involves the immune system. About ten percent of the population may have the type of immune system that can lead to Graves' disease but only a small percent of those individuals ever actually develop hyperthyroidism. This may be due to the fact that they are not exposed to the factors that can trigger this problem. Recent evidence suggests that increased blood levels of cortisone and adrenaline, which may be caused by stress, can affect antibody production by the immune system. However, many patients develop Graves' disease without identifiable stress in their lives. This is another reason for keeping your immune system in the best shape possible.

If you develop Graves' disease it may be several weeks or months before you realize that you are sick. The onset is gradual. The symptoms may be mistaken for simple nervousness due to a stressful life situation or you may be dieting and loosing weight, attributing the weight loss to the diet. That is until the hyperthyroidism has accelerated to excess weight loss, trembling, muscle weakness of the upper arms and thighs and insomnia. Then you may notice an increase in your pulse rate, with episodes of palpitations, increased sweating, and heat intolerance. Your skin may become fine, and hair loss may be noticed as your hair becomes more delicate. Bowel movements may become more frequent. If you are a woman your menstrual flow may lighten and the intervals between menstrual periods may lengthen.

Common signs and symptoms of hyperthyroidism:

Signs	*Symptoms*
Fast heart rate	Palpitations
Trembling hands	Intolerance to heat
Weight loss	Nervousness
Muscle weakness	Insomnia
Warm moist skin	Breathlessness
Hair loss	Increase in bowel movements
Staring	Light or absent menstrual cycles
Enlarged thyroid gland	Fatigue

Graves' disease is also associated with inflammation of the eyes, swelling of the tissues around the eyes, and protrusion of the eyes. The cause of this is unknown at this time and the severity is not related to the degree of thyroid hormone abnormality. Occasionally, patients with Graves' disease develop a lumpy reddish thickening of the skin in front of the shins known as *pretibial myxedema.* This is usually painless and not serious. Again the cause is unknown at this time and the severity is not related to the degree of thyroid hormone abnormality. Also unknown is why this is usually limited to the lower leg or why so few people have it. This disease is treated with antithyroid drugs, Beta-Blocker drugs, radioactive iodine, or surgery. Antithyroid drugs must be monitored closely as they have side effects, one of which can affect your white blood cell count. Beta-Blocker drugs also have their share of side affects so please be sure your doctor monitors these drugs closely.

There is a natural tendency to progress toward hypothyroidism sometimes after you have been hyperthyroid, every patient who has ever had hyperthyroidism due to Graves' disease should have blood tests once a year to measure thyroid function.

The most common thyroid disorder is hypothyroidism. Basically it is caused by an underproduction of thyroid hormone resulting in the slowing down of many bodily functions. The symptoms include fatigue, loss of appetite, inability to tolerate cold, a slow heart rate, weight gain, painful premenstrual periods, fertility problems, muscle weakness, muscle cramps, dry and itchy skin, yellow bumps on the eyelids, hair loss, migraines, hoarseness, respiratory infections, constipation, depression, difficulty concentrating, slow speech, goiter, drooping, swollen eyes. The most common symptoms are fatigue and intolerance to cold. There are also now indications that there is an increase in the sensitivity to many medications.

The thyroid can be affected by poor diet, fluoride in the water, excessive consumption of unsaturated fats, pesticide residues on fruits and vegetables, radiation from x-rays, alcohol and drugs.

The most common disease believed to be the cause of an under active thyroid is called "*Hashimoto's disease*," also called autoimmune or chronic lymphocytic thyroiditis. In this disorder the body becomes allergic to thyroid hormone and produces antibodies against its own thyroid tissue. The immune system produces antibodies that destroy the thyroid. This is the most common thyroid condition in the United States.

Hypothyroidism can be difficult to detect because its often vague signs and symptoms are easily confused with other conditions including the natural aging process, or menopause or even stress and is dismissed as a possible problem. Hypothyroidism affects about 13 million people in the United States, and about 90 percent are women. Women between the ages of thirty and fifty seem to be most prone to this condition. Hashimoto's disease can occur in association with other disorders such as anemia, lupus, yeast infections and rheumatoid arthritis.

The causes for Hypothyroidism vary from radioactive iodine treatment to pituitary problems. Other autoimmune diseases may be associated with this disorder, and other family members may be affected. It may also occur shortly after or many years after the radioactive iodine treatment for hyperthyroidism. This is what happened to me. Spontaneous onset can occur for no apparent reason whatsoever. Hypothyroidism can be related to surgery on the thyroid gland, especially if more than one lobe has been removed. As far as medications go, lithium, high doses of iodine, Amiodarone (a heart medication) can also cause hypothyroidism. Certain resins decrease the absorption of oral thyroid hormone and result in inadequate replacement doses in a patient who is already hypothyroid. A viral infection of the thyroid, which is usually painful, may also be a cause, after a period of hyperthyroidism. In a small percentage of cases it may become permanent. There is also a possibility of hypothyroidism shortly after a pregnancy. The thyroid may go into a period of hyperthyroidism then hypothyroidism then most often it returns to normal. An infant may be born with an inadequate amount of thyroid tissue or an enzyme defect. If this condition is not treated right away, physical and/or mental damage may develop. If there is a history of thyroid problems in the family it may be a good idea to have your baby tested early for any abnormalities. The last known cause at this time is the pituitary hypothyroidism. Any destructive disease of the pituitary gland may cause damage to the cells that stimulate thyroid hormone production. We talked earlier about the pituitary gland and it's relation to the thyroid. There may be other causes, but these are a few to ponder.

Congenital hypothyroidism in children, if left untreated, can lead to mental retardation and dwarfism. A rare condition that can result from long-term undiagnosed hypothyroidism is called *myxedema coma*. The coma can occur during an illness, after an accident or from exposure to cold, or as a result of the ingestion of narcotics and/or sedatives. *This is a medical emergency that requires immediate treatment.*

Treatment for hypothyroidism is to restore normal blood levels of thyroid hormone by replacing it with a synthetic hormone tablet, levothyroxine sodium, which is generally taken for life. Levothyroxine fully replaces thyroid hormone deficiency and can be safely taken for the rest of the patient's life without side effects or complications. However, patient dosage requirements may change over time according to age, body weight, etc., therefore it is essential to monitor patients' medication needs on a regular basis.

Hypothyroid patients *should not switch* to different brands of levothyroxine sodium without consulting his/her physician, according to guidelines set by both the American Association of Clinical Endocrinologists (AACE) and the American Thyroid Association (ATA).

Then we have the condition known as *"Thyroiditis"*. There are three types of this disorder, *"Hashimoto's Thyroiditis,"* *"De Quervain's Thyroiditis,"* and what is called *"Silent Thyroiditis."*

During the course of *Hashimoto's Thyroiditis* the cells of the thyroid become inefficient in converting iodine into thyroid hormone and "compensates" by enlarging. The iodine uptake may be high while the patient is hypothyroid because the gland retains the ability to take-up iodine even after it has lost its ability to produce thyroid hormone. As the disease progresses, the TSH increases since the pituitary is trying to induct the thyroid to make more hormone, the T4 level falls and the patient becomes hypothyroid. This sequence of events can occur over a short span of a few weeks or may take several years. The treatment is to start thyroid hormone replacement. The dosage usually starts slow and is gradually increased. This corrects the hypothyroidism and it also generally keeps the gland from getting larger. Thyroid antibodies may remain for years after the disease has been treated and the patient is on thyroid hormone replacement.

De Quervain's Thyroiditis is much less common, and the thyroid gland generally swells rapidly and is very painful and tender. The gland discharges thyroid hormone into the blood and patients become hyperthyroid. Patients frequently become ill with a fever and are fatigued to the point of wanting to stay in bed. Thyroid antibodies are NOT present in the blood, but the sedimentation rate, which measures inflammation, is very high. Treatment is bed rest and aspirin to reduce inflammation. Occasionally steroids to reduce inflammation and thyroid hormone may be used in prolonged cases. Nearly all patients recover and recurrences are uncommon.

Silent Thyroiditis is the least common type of thyroiditis. Symptoms are similar to Graves Disease except milder, and resembles in part Hashimoto's Thyroiditis and in part De Quervain's Thyroiditis. The blood thyroid tests are high and the iodine uptake is low, but there is no pain. Treatment is usually bed rest with beta-blockers to control palpitations (drugs to prevent rapid heart rates). A few patients have become permanently hypothyroid and have needed to be placed on thyroid hormone permanently.

Testing

Testing

Knowledge of thyroid physiology is important in knowing what thyroid test or tests are needed to diagnose the different thyroid disorders. No single laboratory test is 100% accurate, however, a combination of two or more tests can usually detect even the slightest abnormal thyroid function. For example, if the T4 level is low and the TSH is not elevated, the pituitary gland is more likely to be the cause of hypothyroidism. This would affect the treatment since the pituitary gland also regulates the body's other glands (adrenal, ovaries, and testicles) as well as controlling growth in children and normal kidney function. Pituitary gland failure means that other glands may be failing and treatment other than for the thyroid may be necessary. Listed below are some thyroid function tests and their typical ranges. It is not an exhaustive list.

Thyroid Function Tests

Test	Abbreviation	Typical Ranges
Serum thyroxine	T4	4.6-12 ug/dl
Free thyroxine fraction	FT4F	0.03-0.005%
Free thyroxine	FT4	0.7-1.9 ng/dl
Thyroid hormone binding ratio	THBR	0.9-1.1
Free thyroxine index	FT4I	4-11
Serum Triiodothyronine	T3	80-180 ng/dl
Free Triiodothyronine	FT3	230-619 pg/d

Free T3 index	FT3I	80-180
Radioactive iodine uptake	RAIU	10-30%
Serum thyrotropin	TSH	0.5-6 uU/ml
Thyroxine-binding globulin	TBG	12-20 ug/dl T4 + 1.8 ugm
TRH stimulation test peak	TSH	9-30 uIU/ml at 20-30 min
Serum thyroglobulin	Tg	10-30 ng/m
Thyroid microsomal antibody titer	TMAb	Varies with method
Thyroglobulin antibody titer	TgAb	Varies with method

Since this is not an exhaustive list, there are tests I will mention below that are not on the above chart.

Measurement of Serum Thyroid Hormones ~ T4 by RIA (radio immunoassay). This thyroid test only measures the total T4 and does not correct for certain medications such as birth control pills, seizure medications, cardiac drugs or even aspirin. The FT4 test listed above does correct for this binding procedure. The important point is that T4 is often not adequate. Either FT4I, T7 (which is similar to FT4), or FT4 should be measured.

Measurement of Serum Thyroid Hormone ~ T3 by RIA. Sometimes the thyroid gland will produce high levels of T3 but still produce normal levels of T4, therefore, measurement of both hormones provide an even more accurate evaluation of thyroid function.

Thyroid Binding Globulin ~ This test is not as important any more. Most of the thyroid hormones in the blood are attached to a protein called thyroid-binding globulin (TBG). If there is excess or deficiency of this protein it alters the T4 or T3 measurement, but does not affect the action of the hormone. So if a patient has normal thyroid function, but an unexplained high or low T4, or T3 it may be due to an increase or decrease of TBG. This can cause a false T4 reading. Tests such as the FT4I, T7, and FT4 correct for the changes in the TBG.

Measurement of Pituitary Production of TSH ~ Pituitary production of TSH is measured by a method referred to as IRMA (immunoradiometric assay). Low levels (less than 5 units) of TSH are adequate to keep the normal thyroid gland functioning properly. When the thyroid gland becomes inefficient, the TSH becomes elevated even though the T4 and T3 may be within the "normal" range. The rise in TSH represents the pituitary gland's response to a drop in circulating thyroid hormone. It is usually the first indication of thyroid gland failure. The normally low TSH indicates impaired pituitary function, by failing to rise when circulating thyroid hormones are low. TSH is usually used in combination with other thyroid tests such as those listed above, because interpretation of the TSH level depends on the level of thyroid hormone.

TRH Test ~ this test has become obsolete due to the newer, more sensitive TSH test.

Thyroid Antibodies ~ the body normally produces antibodies to foreign substances in the body; however, some people have antibodies against their own thyroid tissue. The condition known as Hashimoto's Thyroiditis is associated with a high level of these antibodies in the blood. High levels of these antibodies are strong evidence for this disease. Sometimes, low levels of thyroid antibodies are found with other types of thyroid disease. When Hashimoto's Thyroiditis is present as a thyroid nodule rather than a diffuse goiter, the thyroid antibodies may not be present.

The first biopsy/test I had was called an "Ultrasound Guided Needle Biopsy." The technician used the ultrasound to guide the needle into the proper suspicious area of the thyroid gland. This can also give accurate measurements of the nodule's size and if done more than once, can determine whether or not it is growing or shrinking. My doctor at the time told me there was nothing to worry about, that I should take the thyroid hormone therapy, and "we'll see how things go." But, I knew something wasn't right. I still didn't feel well even though they were giving me medication to stabilize my Thyroid Hormone. I had what I called a "yo-yo" effect. Sometimes I was up ~ sometimes I was down. After a year or so of this, I sought out a second opinion. *Never, never, be afraid to get a second opinion! And trust your instincts.*

My new doctor performed another biopsy ~ a "Thyroid Needle Biopsy." In this procedure, which was done in the doctor's office, a needle is inserted into the thyroid gland to take out tissue, sometimes from several areas. I was able to return to my normal routine right afterwards. No anesthesia is required for this procedure. It was not comfortable, but bearable as my focus was on getting an answer for my symptoms. The pathologist's report showed "atypical cells" and "Hurthle cells". My doctor told me, both are suspicious when it comes to diagnosing cancer. It was at that point that I began to prepare myself mentally. The cancer diagnosis had not been fully made, but I prepared for the worst leaning on my faith to stabilized me and keep me grounded in truth. It is so easy to let the mind just go and when it does stress usually results. I didn't want to deal with more than was necessary at the time.

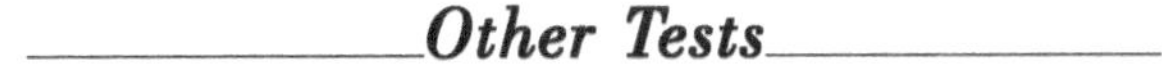

Other Tests

Thyroid Scan ~ Produces a picture of the thyroid taken after a small dose of radioactive iodine has been swallowed. The scan visualizes the thyroid and the nodule. It also shows whether the nodule is functioning or not. A functioning nodule is sometimes referred to as a "hot" nodule, and a nonfunctioning nodule is sometimes referred to as a "cold" nodule. Cancer is rarely found in a "hot" nodule. If a "hot" nodule causes hyperthyroidism, it can be treated with radioiodine. Most thyroid scans show that thyroid nodules are "cold." This does not mean that the nodule is cancerous, but it does mean that further evaluation is needed. If this applies to you please don't let it sit too long.

Thyroid Needle Biopsy ~ We touched on this one earlier. The test is not perfect, however, it will provide a diagnosis in more than seventy five percent of the biopsy specimens. This drastically reduces the number of patients who have to undergo operations for benign nodules. About twenty percent are interpreted as inconclusive, meaning that the pathologist can't be certain the nodule is cancerous. Your physician can use other criteria to make a decision about the need to operate. These inconclusive biopsies are usually repeated with the use of the thyroid ultrasonography.

Thyroid Ultrasonography ~ The most important use of the thyroid ultrasonography is in aiding the guiding of the biopsy needle to obtain a sample from the solid portion of the nodule or nodules, and avoiding specimens from surrounding normal thyroid tissue, especially if the nodule is small in size. The thyroid ultrasound also provides an objective and precise method for detecting changes in the nodule's size. A nodule that is stable and not increasing in size usually does not require surgical treatment.

There may be newer tests now that I am not aware of as of this writing, so please ask questions as to which test is most reliable for your symptoms.

Cancer

Cancer

Without a doubt it is the most dreaded word in the English language, a word that can strike fear into the heart of any family. Cancer brings us face to face with the sharp realization of our mortality and a fight for life. Cancer no matter what the type is a life long condition and affects our entire family.

Thyroid cancer, though it has a high cure and low return rate, is a cancer that you live with every day for the rest of your life. It is a cancer that is not often talked about, and/or written about. Rarely does it make headlines. But to you and me this is serious business.

Thyroid Cancers

Most people with thyroid cancer have a growth or lump that has gradually grown, in the thyroid gland. Usually no symptoms are present except the lump in the neck that may cause a feeling of pressure. In most cases the lump is painless. Any lump or uncomfortable feeling should be reported to your physician immediately! There are several types of thyroid cancer as I mentioned earlier.

Papillary Carcinoma (This is the one I had). It is the most common thyroid cancer. Papillary tumors make up about seventy to eighty percent of all thyroid cancers, and can occur at any age. It usually occurs in only one lobe of the thyroid, but both lobes are involved ten to twenty percent of the time. It is often associated with a history of radiation exposure and spreads through the *lymphatics*. There can also be a genetic predisposition for this type of cancer. Even though papillary cancer grows slowly, it often spreads early to the lymph nodes in the neck. Patients with papillary carcinoma who have a primary tumor that is intrathyroidal (confined to the thyroid gland itself) have an excellent outlook; the twenty-five year mortality rate from cancer in this situation is about one percent. This means that only one out of every one hundred such patients have died of thyroid cancer by twenty-five years later. By that time the vast majority of them have been permanently cured. The prognosis is not quite as good in patients over the age of fifty, or in patients with tumors larger than four centimeters (1 ½ inches) in diameter. Nor is it as good in patients where the cancer has grown through the thyroid into surrounding tissues. Specifically, through the fibrous capsule that surrounds the thyroid gland into the tissues of the neck. In a very small percentage of patients (about five percent), the cancer spreads through the blood stream to distant sites, particularly the lungs and bones. Surgery is almost always curative when the thyroid gland is totally or nearly totally removed. Radiation treatment follows when you reach the state of being *hypothyroid*. Repeat treatments may be required every six to twelve months, depending on the extent of the cancer. Slightly higher doses than the normal dose of *thyroid hormone* are given after the surgery and treatment, which may make you slightly hyperthyroid for the rest of your life.

Follicular Thyroid Cancer develops in the structures of the thyroid gland called by that name. This is the second most common type of thyroid cancer and is also called *follicular cancer*, *follicular carcinoma*, or *follicular adenocarcinoma*. These cancers usually stay in the thyroid gland but can spread to other parts of the body, such as lungs and bone. *Follicular carcinomas* do not often spread to lymph nodes, but when they do the lymph nodes are removed during surgery. The same treatment is given for this type of cancer as for the *Papillary Carcinoma*.

Medullary Thyroid Cancer, can occur at any age and may be part of a familial syndrome called *Multiple Endocrine Neoplasia Type II*. In families with *MEN II*, genetic testing can be performed to identify affected members. This is the only thyroid cancer that develops from the *C-cells* of the thyroid gland. This cancer can spread to the lymph nodes, the lungs, or liver even before a thyroid nodule is discovered or a screening test is done. This cancer usually makes *calcitonin* and *carcinoembryonic antigen (CEA)*. *Calcitonin* is a hormone produced by normal *C-cells* that help control the amount of calcium in the blood. Both *calcitonin* and *CEA* are released into the blood and can be detected by blood tests. This too can be treated by surgically removing the entire thyroid unless the cancer has spread to another part of the body. If it has spread then chemotherapy will be added. Also removed are any lymph nodes that contain the cancer since they can cause the spreading of it to other parts of the body.

Anaplastic Carcinoma is a rare form of thyroid cancer. It is believed to develop from an existing papillary or follicular cancer. This tumor grows rapidly and painfully, often invading the neck and other parts of the body. About eighty percent of the patients die within one year of the diagnosis. The treatment is quick and the total thyroid as well as surrounding tissue is removed. Because this type of thyroid cancer spreads quickly to other tissues it is not uncommon for the patient to lose some of the trachea (the tube through which a person breathes). External radiation therapy and chemotherapy accompany the above. Some clinical trials are now in existence for this type of thyroid cancer.

Thyroid Lymphoma can develop in the thyroid gland but is very uncommon in that location. Lymphomas develop from *lymphocytes*, the main cell type of the immune system. Most are found in pea-sized clusters scattered throughout the body in the lymph nodes. This type of thyroid cancer causes the immune system to attack the person's own thyroid gland. This results in many *lymphocytes* in the thyroid gland. If the cancer has not spread beyond the thyroid it can be treated with surgery or radiation therapy. If the cancer has spread, chemotherapy, with or without radiation therapy is used.

Your doctor will have more details on these types of cancer, most specifically, your type of cancer. The above information is just an overview, not a complete fact sheet about the cancer or the treatments.

Treatments

Treatments

Treatments for thyroid cancer include surgery, radioactive iodine treatment, thyroid hormone therapy, external beam radiation therapy, and chemotherapy. Surgery is the most common treatment for cancer of the thyroid.

> *Lobectomy* removes only the side of the thyroid where the cancer is found. Lymph nodes in the area may be taken out for biopsy to see if they contain cancer.
> *Near-total thyroidectomy*, as the name implies, nearly removes the entire thyroid.
> *Total thyroidectomy*—I had this surgery—removes the entire thyroid.
> *Lymph node dissection* removes cancer-containing lymph nodes in the neck.

Anesthetic is given and you will be asleep during the operation. You can expect to be ready to leave the hospital in three to seven days. Some potential complications of thyroid surgery include temporary or permanent hoarseness or voice loss (if nerves are damaged), damage to the parathyroid glands (small glands near the thyroid that help regulate calcium levels in the blood), excessive bleeding, and wound infection. When most of the thyroid is removed, part of the strategy for treating thyroid cancer is to have the patient take thyroid hormone pills after surgery. You may also need extra calcium supplements if your parathyroids were upset during surgery.

Radiation Therapy uses high-energy x-rays to kill cancer cells and shrink tumors. Radiation may come from a machine outside the body or from drinking a liquid that contains radioactive iodine.

External Beam Radiation Therapy uses high-energy rays to destroy cancer cells or slow their rate of growth. A carefully focused beam is delivered from a machine outside the body. The main drawback to this method is that the radiation can also destroy nearby healthy tissue along with the cancer cells; fatigue is another potential side effect. This treatment option can involve treatments five days a week for about six weeks.

Radioactive Iodine Therapy can destroy the thyroid gland and the cancer without affecting the rest of the body. Because the thyroid takes up iodine, the radioactive iodine collects in any thyroid tissue remaining in the body and kills the cancer cells. For this to have the most effect you must have a high thyroid stimulating hormone (TSH) level in the blood. This means discontinuing your thyroid hormone pills one to two weeks before the treatment. This causes a condition known as *hypothyroidism*, which means that your thyroid hormone levels are very low. Side effects of this treatment are rare, but include neck tenderness, nausea and stomach irritation, irritation of the gastrointestinal tract or the bladder, tenderness in the salivary glands, and dry mouth. This therapy is not used to treat Anaplastic and Medullary thyroid carcinomas. (I had the radioactive iodine treatment)

Hypothyroidism has some side effects you should know about. You may feel run down, slow, sluggish, and tired. You may feel cold and depressed. You may loose interest in day-to-day activities. You may have dry brittle hair, dry itchy skin, and constipation, muscle cramps and if that's not enough, you may experience mental dullness. For women there is the chance of increased menstrual flow. We touched on these symptoms earlier.

THYROGEN (thyrotropin alfa for injection) is like the thyroid stimulating hormone (TSH) that your body produces naturally, although it is made in a laboratory.

There is a new procedure using THYROGEN. This allows you to stay on your thyroid hormone therapy and still go through the screening process or the surgery. THYROGEN is a huge blessing in that there is no down time from the thyroid hormone therapy. No missed work, no re-adjustment period for your body once you get back on the therapy. No getting sick with all of the hypothyroid symptoms.

The THYROGEN procedure is only good when you are doing well. If your risk for cancer recurrence is high, you may need to test again while you are off the thyroid hormone therapy. And that is definite when your tests show that you need radioactive iodine treatment.

The Genzyme Corporation and the Knoll Pharmaceutical Company have a brochure, often displayed in doctors' offices, about this alternative preparation. Please ask your doctor about this and be informed.

Hormone Therapy is used to replace the thyroid hormone that is needed after a thyroidectomy and also to decrease the TSH levels that can stimulate thyroid growth. My first doctor used this therapy to try to reduce the size of the nodule and my thyroid. However this was unsuccessful.

Chemotherapy uses drugs to kill cancer cells. It may be taken as a pill or it may be put into the body by a needle in the vein of a muscle. Chemotherapy is called a systemic treatment because the drug enters the bloodstream and can kill cancer cells outside the thyroid.

There is a product known as *714X* that has been instrumental in the treatment and cure of autoimmune or degenerative diseases, including cancer. 714X makes no distinction between types of cancer, since it works on your natural defenses, more precisely on your immune system. There is a protocol that the manufacturer recommends and I suggest that, as an alternative to the common treatment, you get more information on this particular treatment for thyroid cancer. 714X is an immunomodulator and has been used in Canada since January 1990, as an Emergency Drug. The Canadian Government has given over 17,000 authorizations for 714X. In the resource section of this book, I will include information on how to contact the company. There is a wealth of information on their website and they are more than willing to help with additional information. This is worth looking into as an alternative to radiation and chemotherapy, or it could be a complementary treatment, depending on one's personal choice. 714X is a health product used in a variety of diseases including thyroid cancer. (The FDA in the United States has not yet approved this product.)

Please use all of the resources at your disposal to get all the information you can on your particular type of thyroid cancer and on your particular type of treatment or treatments if you need more than one.

Can I Be Patient?

Can I Be Patient?

It has been said that "Patience is a virtue," but I have to say that patience is a blessing. We all have some, at least for some things. We can wait patiently for our child to be born because we have a due date. We can wait patiently for that new car when we know we are going to get it soon. But with cancer, there is no due date; there is no assurance that this will be over soon. So, you may be wondering why I called patience a blessing. Well, read on.

Once the diagnosis is made, you want to get to the treatment. What do I have to do and how fast can we do this? Now is the time for patience ~ patience with your doctor and patience with yourself ~ are of the utmost importance at this stage. This is when you take a step back, talk about and ask about the cancer and your treatment options. And remember, you are not the only one affected. Cancer, as I mentioned before, is a family condition. It will also be with you for the rest of your life. Patience is **IMPORTANT.**

The "doing" of patience is the true blessing. If you can do the above, waiting for answers, searching out your best treatment options, and planning. All of this is part of being patient, and I know you can do this. If I can, anyone can. It did take some forethought, realizing that I was not in control, nor could I ever be in control. I could however take responsibility, which lead to patience. I had to take responsibility for my health and my cancer. It was, after all mine.

Please try to be patient, and do the things that lead to patience. You will have much less stress and some input into what happens to you. Even if you are not in control, you can contribute.

I am including a list of questions to ask and discuss with your doctor. After that there are several pages for you to write notes and answers to these VERY IMPORTANT questions.

| *Questions*

Questions

There are questions that you will want to ask first, and questions someone else will want to ask first. The following questions are not in any specific order, therefore it's up to you to decide what is most important to you and start there. There is space to write in your own questions at the end of each section. I know that I may not have covered everything. Each of us is different and we each have individual needs and in this case questions.

_______*Questions about the cancer*_______

- ✼ What type of cancer do I have? (Please get the specifics)
- ✼ Has this cancer or tumor invaded the thyroid gland, the lymphatic system, or has it been introduced into the blood stream?
- ✼ Is there cancer in both sides of my thyroid gland?
  There were suspicious cells in both sides of my thyroid gland and my surgeon opted to take the entire thing out. I strongly believe in "if in doubt ~ take it all out." There are those who will disagree, but you and your doctor will make that final decision. Make sure it is an informed one.
- ✼ Has my cancer spread to other parts of my body? (Again ask for specifics)
- ✼ Can you tell from the tests the size of the nodule or tumor?
- ✼ How far has my cancer progressed, what stage am I in?
- ✼ Is this type of cancer hereditary, should my family be tested?
- ✼ If not, can you tell me what caused my cancer? (Most of the time there is no answer to this question ~ but sometimes there is ~ SO ASK.)
- ✼ Other:
- ✼ Other:
- ✼ Other:

Some of these questions won't lend themselves to answers until after the surgery when the pathology report is in. *Please be patient with your self and your doctor.*

______*Questions about the surgery*______

Since surgery is the most common treatment this is an important step. Your endocrinologist will recommend a surgeon to you. Contacting the surgeon and meeting with him/her is a very important interview. I had a fabulous surgeon and I pray you will have the same. If you are not comfortable, don't hesitate to ask your doctor to recommend someone else for you. The surgery is difficult enough without being uncomfortable with someone who will literally cut on your body.

- Do I need to have the entire thyroid gland removed or just a portion? *(Total thyroidectomy Vs. partial thyroidectomy)*
- What are the pros and cons of each?
- If only a partial is done, will a biopsy be done on the other side?
- What happens if only a partial is done and the pathologist suspects cancer on the other side?
- How long before I face surgery again? (If the previous question applies to you.)
- What are the possible risks/side effects/complications of the surgery?
- What is the exact procedure that will be used on me?
- Where will the incision be made and how large will the scar be?
- How long does this procedure usually take, and how long will I be under anesthesia?
- What can I expect when I wake up after surgery? (I had a huge ice pack on my neck when I wakened, and it stayed on for quite some time)
- How long will I be in the hospital after the surgery?
- If I need treatment, how long will it be between the surgery and the treatment?
- When can I return to work?
- Other:
- Other:
- Other:

______*Questions about your treatment*______

- What type of treatment is required for the type of cancer I have?
- What is the recommended time between surgery and treatment?
- Do I need the type of radiation treatment that requires an oral dose of radioactive iodine?
- If so, how large of a dose will I receive?
- What preparations do I need to make in order to have this type of treatment?
- If radioactive iodine kills cancer cells what will it do to the rest of my body?
- What are the specific complications and side effects of my type of radiation therapy?
- How long will I be in the hospital with this type of radiation treatment and what does that hospital stay require?
- After I am released from the hospital, will I have to take precautions because of having radiation?

Having had the Radioactive Iodine Treatment, I was very unprepared for the hospital stay and the specific requirements and restrictions when it was time for me to go home. The following is some very important information regarding radioactive iodine treatment. The required dosage for hospitalization is now 200mCi. However at the time of my treatment the dosage required for hospitalization was 100mCi. For those who have less than the 200mCi units of radiation, you will go home with some of the same restrictions that were required of me. The restrictions will be slightly altered and there will be additional restrictions.

If you require hospitalization you will be in what I called the "plastic room." You can't take much into the room because it becomes contaminated with the radiation in your body. Everything was covered in new plastic ~ the floor, ceiling, bed, telephone, etc. While I was in there I had a problem with nausea from the smell of the plastic. And if it happens to you don't hesitate to make yourself comfortable, at least as comfortable as possible. There are shots you can take for the nausea. ASK YOUR NURSE!

Many showers (about three or four a day) during the treatment while you are in the hospital helps to pass the time and pass the radiation from your system. You are not going to want to do that, because you are tired. However, sleep, eat, drink plenty of water, and SHOWER, and soon you will be able to go home. A good book is always a plus to pass the time. There will be no visitors. Even the nurses can't be around your level of radiation for any length of time. Up to three days in the hospital is normal. To limit the contamination of personal items, you should bring only what you will need. Your clothing should be limited to what you were wearing when admitted. Try to bring only paperback books, magazines, and newspapers instead of hard cover books, craft items, or work related items.

To minimize the effect of the radioactive iodine on your salivary glands; suck on sour lemon drops or lemon slices for the first day or so. This too is very important.

Be prepared for the scores of limitations you will have when you get home. Ask about them right away, not just before you go home. I'll touch on some here.

Your family should prepare for you to come home to a semi-secluded environment to reduce exposure to others. The amount of exposure to others will depend on how long you are with them and at what distance they are from you. Someone two feet away will receive only one fourth of the exposure as someone only one foot away.

For the first two to three days you should use only one restroom in your home (if that is possible). Flush the toilet two or three times after each use. Bathe every day and of course wash your hands often. You should drink normal amounts of fluids. Try to use disposable eating utensils. If at all possible, sleep alone and avoid prolonged intimate contact. You should launder your own items separately, including any towels or linens you use. (Nothing special needs to be done to your washing machine or dryer between your loads and the loads of items from other members of the family.) DO NOT prepare food that requires you to use your bare hands.

For the next five days after your treatment your doctor or radiation technician may recommend continued precautions depending on the amount of radiation you received.

The radiation department will give you a list of "don't do's" that include some of the ones mentioned above. Make sure you **ask** if there are any other precautions you should take, especially if you have small children. The new regulations are not as confining as the ones I had and they will probably change again, **but to adhere to the restrictions is crucial.**

You will go back to the hospital to have your levels checked for safe limits before all goes back to normal. For me it was seven days. For some people it takes less time, for others it takes longer.

Again I remind you to please **ask** about what your family needs to do *before* you get home. It isn't worth contaminating your kids just because it is difficult to have restrictions at home. This too shall pass! Let your friends and family help you, let them cook for you, let them come and clean your house, let them do your laundry, etc.

_____*Now back to the questions*_____

- ❧ When can I expect to return to work?
- ❧ Will this treatment affect my ability to bear children?
- ❧ If not, how long do I need to avoid getting pregnant?
- ❧ If I need external beam radiation, what side effects should I expect?
- ❧ Will I have a hospital stay with this type of treatment?
- ❧ What is the recovery time for this type of treatment?
- ❧ As with the radioactive iodine treatment, what will happen to the cells that aren't cancerous?
- ❧ How many treatments do I need?
- ❧ Do I need chemotherapy?
- ❧ What are the side effects of this type of treatment?
- ❧ What can I do to minimize the side effects of chemotherapy?
- ❧ How many treatments will I have to have?
- ❧ What is the recovery time with chemotherapy?
- ❧ Can I work while having this/these chemotherapy treatments?
- ❧ Again, will this treatment affect my ability to bear children?
- ❧ Again, if not, how long should I wait before getting pregnant?
- ❧ Do I have to have more than one of these treatments?
- ❧ If so, what can I expect, and what is my part in the treatment schedule?
- ❧ What other treatment choices do I have?
- ❧ Other:
- ❧ Other:
- ❧ Other:

You will meet with the treatment department technicians and doctors. Please question them also. They are the ones who actually perform the procedures and can be more than helpful if you have any questions or concerns on the day/days of your treatment. The nurses assigned to you when you have a hospital stay are also very informed. The radiation department and the chemotherapy departments are two departments you must question thoroughly!

_____*Questions about recurrence*_____

- ❧ What are the chances that my cancer will recur?
- ❧ What symptoms should I look for?
- ❧ How and when will I be screened for a recurrence of this cancer?

- If there is a recurrence, in what part of the body does my type of cancer usually recur?
- For how many years after the treatment is recurrence possible?
- If my cancer does come back, will the treatment be the same?
- Will there be other doctors who will follow my case long-term?

___Questions about hormone replacement___

- Will I need thyroid hormone replacement therapy for the rest of my life?
- Which doctor will be prescribing this for me?
- Which doctor will monitor the levels of the hormone in my body?
- What symptoms will I have while the proper level for me is being determined?
- How and how often will my hormone levels be checked?
- How will over-the-counter prescriptions interact with the other drugs I am taking?
- What are the side effects of the thyroid hormone therapy?
- Other:
- Other:
- Other:
- And the question on everyone's mind ~

> ***Based on all the information about my thyroid cancer what is my chance of survival and how long do you think I will survive?***

*You don't have to have answers to all of these questions right away. Remember patience. Your cancer is a process. You **did not** get it overnight and **it won't go away** overnight. **Patience.** Allow your doctor time to answer or find answers to all of your questions. **Patience.**

Notes

Notes

This is the section for notes you may want to take when you are talking to the doctors, and other medical personnel as well jotting down the answers to the questions we went over.

____

____

____

____

____

____

____

____

____

The Preparation

The Preparation

Prepare for change. Everything will change. The way you look at life will change. The way you look at yourself and your family will change. Your priorities will change. Your eating habits *must* change. Your mind *must* change, because excuses for not changing come easily. "It's too hard," "I can't afford the food or supplements, I can't cook, I can't . . ." It is very easy to get a case of the "I cant's." Be ready for change. Be ready for your whole world to change. However this is not the time to become overwhelmed. The changes will come slowly and steadily and with this book and other resources, hopefully you will be more prepared.

Prepare for health! We did not get cancer over night and we will not get well overnight. Getting healthy is a process. We have to prepare with the proper information about how to get this health we so desire. Take the time to get started on preparing for all this. We will focus on preparing our mind in the next section. Now we will concentrate on preparing for health.

Once the diagnosis of cancer has been made we want to rush into the treatment immediately. Certainly you don't want to delay, especially if you have Anaplastic carcinoma, however, there is one **very important** factor that needs your attention. **Your immune system;** it is and has been taking a beating, because your immune system has been fighting thyroid cancer for who knows how long. *Preparing yourself and your family* is a very important part of dealing with cancer. Therefore, find out from your doctor how long you can wait before you need the treatment.

Prepare your body. At the risk of repeating myself, let me again emphasize your need to concentrate on your immune system. No matter what type of cancer you have or what type of treatment you have, there must be time to prepare your body. You must be sure your immune system is in the best shape possible both to minimize the damage of the treatment on your body, and to minimize the side effects. And most importantly you don't want to have to deal with another cancer **from the treatment.** Stay informed about your treatment. Excluding nutritional therapy, the treatments all have side effects that can **cause cancer,** and surgery has it's own risks.

Prepare yourself and your family. Since all you will go through will affect your entire family it is important to share all information concerning your condition with your family. Smaller children will be harder to share with, however, they too will feel the changes around them. Inform your family of food and lifestyle changes you intend to make and get their input. Some of the changes may only benefit you. And most certainly they will not go on the low-iodine diet with you. And please, please, inform your family of the procedures before coming home from any radiation or chemotherapy treatment.

Also, you will want to do most of your food shopping and planning ahead of time. Make up menus of allowed foods. Shop ahead of time. Prepare as much of the food as you can ahead of time. When you are hypothyroid from lack of hormone you will not want to do some of the things that you planned to do. You will be too sick and tired. Breads can be baked and frozen ahead of time; snacks can also be prepared, as can many meals. Begin to prepare as soon as possible, before you are just too tired. The secret is early preparation!

The Immune System

The Immune System

Let's briefly discuss the immune system. Of what does it consist? Why is it so necessary for you to make it a priority?

You really are what you eat! In addition to your body's built-in, natural immune system, it also has an energy factory. The first step toward improved health is to eat fresh, clean foods. Digestion begins in the mouth, moves to the stomach, then to the small intestine. If your system isn't working properly, some detoxification and cleansing may be required. Discuss the process with a nutritionist and/or your doctor. There are many books and pamphlets on cleansing and detoxification. Check with your doctor before you do any cleansing and/or detoxification.

Your ability to digest these healthy foods and supplements is crucial to your achieving a healthy body. If we can't digest and distribute the nutrients from the good things we eat we are not taking enough forward steps. Again, go over this with your doctor and/or a nutritionist.

Your body has built-in defenders that defend against sickness and disease. Your immune system is a complex system.

There is the ***lymphatic system*** that consists of vessels and organs.

The ***tonsils*** in the back of our throat produce antibodies that help fight bacteria that cause infections.

The ***liver*** where white blood cells are produced helps remove organisms from the blood as it passes through, acting as a "filter."

The ***mucous membranes*** in the respiratory and gastrointestinal tracts repel organisms and allergens. They also battle against any organisms that try to penetrate them.

New white blood cells grow up and develop specialized functions in the *thymus.*

The *spleen* removes abnormal cells from circulation.

The *lymph* nodes act as filters and produce antibodies to destroy invading organisms and abnormal cells.

The *skin* keeps organisms and allergens from entering the body. (Keeping cuts and scrapes to a minimum during this time is important).

The *white blood cells;* lymphocytes, neutrophils, basophils, eosinophils, monocytes; are specialized cells that reside in various tissues and in specialized serum factors.

The *thymus* is the master gland of the immune system. It lies just below the thyroid gland and above the heart. It is extremely susceptible to free-radical damage caused by stress, drugs, radiation, infection and chronic illness; therefore it undergoes shrinkage, as we grow older. The *thymus* is responsible for many immune system functions. It produces white blood cells called *"T lymphocytes."* It is responsible for what is called *"cell-mediated immunity," a* process extremely important in resisting infections by mold like bacteria, yeast, fungi, parasites, and viruses. Cell-mediated immunity is critical in protecting against the development of cancer and allergies. Fresh juice can be helpful in prevention of thymus shrinkage, in acting as a cofactor for thymic hormones and in stimulating thymus activity. Juicing alone cannot do that if you are seriously ill. To keep the thymus healthy, herbs, nutritional supplements, special nutritional factors and other supportive therapies are necessary. Some of which we will discuss in this book.

Everything we do has a major impact on our body's immune system. It is important to go into this battle fully armed with the healthiest diet and nutrition program possible so that you will have the best chance of successfully conquering cancer. I'd like to start by getting your immune system ready for the battle ahead. There are many things you can do. The best, of course, is proper nutrition. A good nutritionist is worth his/her weight in gold. Remember it is your immune system that needs your attention first. With very few exceptions, side effects such as weight gain or loss, hair loss, mood swings, may have to be dealt with later.

Two underlying conditions that could hinder all your hard work in getting healthy and fighting this cancer are Candida and parasites. Candida is a common yeast found in the body. Sometimes it starts to grow out of control. This can be caused by repeated antibiotic use, birth control pills, too much sugar, high progesterone, vaginal yeast, unfiltered water, undercooked foods, pets, and sometimes travel outside of the US.

Parasites are mostly microscopic. Sometimes however, they are hookworms, roundworms, and pinworms. They coexist well with yeast. Indicators of parasites include: *Persistent Bloating & Gas ~ Diarrhea ~ Constipation ~ Joint and Muscle Pain ~ Allergies ~ Chronic Bowel Irritation ~ Chronic Fatigue ~ Skin Disorders ~ Insomnia ~ Brain Fog ~ Food Sensitivities ~ Bad Breath ~ Burning Urination ~ and Sugar Cravings.* If you have any of these symptoms you may have to undergo a cleansing as a first step to getting healthy. You must make sure that your body can and will properly digest the nutrients you give it and that you are therefore getting the maximum benefits. Again, cleansing must be done under the care of a physician and/or nutritionist.

At the end of this book I will list some helpful resources, but I'll recommend some things here in a general way to help you get started on your path to better health and to help get you started on boosting your immune system for the treatment ahead. We need good nutrition, rest, exercise and even sunlight. It's hard work, but well worth the benefits. What's harder than going through cancer anyway?

We need to take care of our body's defenses. We need to limit our exposure to anyone who is sick and to germs and viruses. Washing our hands often.

Let's start with some harmful things to cut completely out of our diet and our life during this time, and then get to some things that we can add to our diet and our life.

<>< Sugar! **What,** you say? Yes, *refined* sugar cripples the immune system. It actually coats the cells so that they become virtually useless to us. It takes over four hours for sugar to wear off of your good cells. We need them, let's not hinder them.

<>< STAY AWAY FROM MSG. It is found in virtually all processed foods, even the ones that say they are MSG-free. The government allows a certain amount ~ an amount that they call safe ~ to be used.

<>< Caffeine is a toxin in your body, especially now.

<>< Alcohol dehydrates your body.

<>< Solid fat stays solid in your system; liquid fat stays liquid in your system. I mean fat at room temperature. So limit your meat and solid fats.

<>< Stay away from artificial sweeteners. Unfortunately they are found in over 1600 food products, so watch what you buy.

<>< I don't think I have to tell you what smoking does to your immune system so I won't go into that. The dangers of smoking and second hand smoke are advertised sufficiently.

<>< Chlorine as well as fluoride, is harmful to the body. These chemicals are supposed to keep the water clean and help protect your teeth, however, they are chemicals you don't need right now, actually that you never need. You should always avoid these toxins. You can have your water checked or you can opt for better drinking water using filtration systems or faucet filters.

<>< Dehydration. We can very easily become dehydrated long before we ever get thirsty. **Drink water.** Drink bottled, purified or distilled water, PLEASE! The body also needs water in order to flush toxins from your body. If you don't drink enough they just stay there and you can't afford that risk now. Again let me add here that chlorine and fluoride are toxic to the body so please drink purified, distilled or at least filtered water, and lots of it.

<>< Stress is one of the greatest factors in suppressing the immune system. Right now you are undergoing much stress just from the diagnosis of this cancer. There are stress busters that can help. Pull out your Bible and start de-stressing! Have a greater understanding and awareness of your body, be free of negative thoughts that drain your energy, and replace them with strengthened mental and spiritual balance. There are a variety of other resources that your doctor can recommend. My preference is the Bible.

<>< Studies have indicated that a high-fat diet increases the risk of cancer, while a low-fat diet that is rich in fiber, fresh fruit, vegetables, and whole grains actually help the body fight cancer.

<>< Nervous energy and stress deplete the immune system of essential nutrients such as B vitamins. Ask your doctor about a supplement if you are a nervous person or if you have stresses beyond the cancer.

<>< The most overlooked factor and the most often ignored is exercise. Exercise! Yes, that's what I said. Who feels like exercising when it takes everything you have to get out of bed? As I stated before, you want to prepare for this battle so you can fare well through it all and continue a healthy lifestyle afterward. *Cancer is less prevalent in physically active people.* Exercise also helps prevent depression and promotes oxygenation of tissue.

It has been said that exercise is the closest thing to a "magic bullet" when it comes to optimal health and well being when combined with a well-balanced diet. Set down a program that is right for you and meets with your doctor's approval. Do what you can and increase, as you are able. Here are some tips for people undergoing cancer treatments.

** Choose activities that are comfortable, accessible and enjoyable, with stretching and relaxation at each session. Try a variety of different exercises; choose the ones that give you the most benefit without wearing you out.

** Walking is a simple way to begin; it can boost your spirit as well as your immune system. It can also decrease fatigue and aid in recovery. Once or twice every other day, starting with five to ten minutes.

** On your better days exercise a little longer, on days you feel very tired, do a shorter routine and make sure you stretch.

** Check with your doctor to see if there are exercise programs that are specifically designed for cancer patients in your area. Some area hospitals or rehab centers are now making these programs available. This will help keep you motivated.

Exercise is *extremely important*: don't get discouraged. Again, there are many resources your doctor can recommend. Your doctor will let you know for sure what is right for you.

<>< Along with exercise, rest is essential to your health. Our bodies heal during our sleep cycles. The interval between sundown and midnight contains the prime healing hours. Don't discard the rest of the night though and even naps during the day can be beneficial.

<>< Take some time each day to play and enjoy your family and friends. That too will enhance your immune system and have benefits that cannot be described in words.

<>< I believe that sunlight is also a direct boost to the immune system. Not only does it help prevent stress, it is also a factor in turning cholesterol into vitamins that are helpful to the immune system. Natural sunlight through the eyes goes into the part of the brain that produces Melatonin. (*This does **NOT** mean looking directly into the sun.*) And that center produces hormones that control the immune system. So once in a while sit outside (moderately of course). And on cloudy days, take off your sunglasses and give your immune system a good boost.

Now that you have cancer it is very important to maintain a good healthy immune system and maintain overall health. You may feel that I'm repeating myself, but I want to get the point across to you that a healthy immune system isn't just important now, it will be for the rest of your life.

Just as we all *look* different, our bodies are different. What one person reacts well to, another may become ill from. That is why treatments prove to be successful for some but not for others. It is the reason dietary wellness and prevention is so important. If we keep our bodies healthy and avoid known cancer-causing agents, we can help defend against fighting cancer again.

When you have cancer your whole body is sick! I'll repeat that. **WHEN YOU HAVE CANCER YOUR WHOLE BODY IS SICK.**

Lets go over some nutritional "dos" and "can's" that will help you understand what you can do to boost your immune system.

- <><   There are certain foods that help to fight cancer. These include broccoli, Brussels sprouts, cabbage, cauliflower, and spinach.
- <><   Also carrots, pumpkin, squash, and yams are in this group.
- <><   Apples, berries (including blueberries, raspberries, and strawberries), cantaloupes, cherries, grapes, oranges, and plums are great cancer busters. Berries help protect DNA from damage.
- <><   Also helpful are Brazil nuts, legumes (including chick peas, lentils, and red beans), and almonds are very helpful (about 10 a day).
- <><   Onions and garlic as well as red and yellow peppers are helpful.
- <><   Fresh juice is also very important and we will do some juicing. It is best to consume your fruit juice in the morning and your vegetable juice in the afternoon.

There are many more can's and do's that we will go into when I talk about the "low-iodine." Preparing your body for the treatment of this cancer is as important if not more important than preparing your mind.

Perseverance

Perseverance

Having thyroid cancer and the radiation treatment and being off the thyroid hormone for literally months, has given me this strong desire to encourage those who are going through this ordeal.

Preparing your mind is important and perseverance plays a large part in it.

Denial is a very hindering mindset. We tell ourselves that we eat well. We exercise, we do what we think are all the right things. However, we have cancer. Take responsibility for your cancer. And don't be afraid to ask the tough questions about how this could happen to you. You just might get an answer. I did.

Deciding to be healthy is a choice. Make the decision now, before going on with the rest of the book. And do go on with the rest of the book even if you are skeptical.

You now know about your cancer. You now know about the treatment. You now know about the immune system. Now it's decision-making time. What worked for me, may not work for you. You may have to do some things differently. The things in this book are fairly universal, but there are always exceptions. You have to decide now, that you want to get healthy and you have to know why! The biggest hindrance to change is that it takes time and commitment.

To change according to Webster's Ninth New Collegiate Dictionary, means to "make radically different," "to give a different position, course or direction, to replace with another." It means that we have to do something. Change is an action, and change takes perseverance.

Perseverance starts, but does not end here. Actually perseverance doesn't end at all. It is a beginning that can carry you through with a positive attitude and a positive outlook.

According to Webster's, to persevere means "to persist in a state, enterprise, or undertaking in spite of counter influences, opposition, or discouragement."

It is said to be "the action or condition or an instance of persevering; steadfastness." It means to do something.

I emphasize perseverance at this stage because things will get hard, you will get discouraged, you will feel helpless, and sometimes hopeless. My prayer is that when those times hit you, and they will, you will remember to persevere.

You are not the only one with thyroid cancer. You are not alone. You are not alone in your feelings, your anger or in various other reactions that accompany this diagnosis. All of the things you will go through will pass in time. Perseverance will take you through them all. The Thyca Corporation has resources to find support groups in your area. If there isn't one, maybe it's time to make another change in your life and add this to your list of things to do. I will give more information on the Thyca Corporation in a later section.

One thing at a time, one day at a time. That was my motto. I said those words over and over to myself many times. Especially when my mind would go into its "think too much" mode. Don't try to figure out tomorrow and don't think about yesterday. Concentrate on today! Tomorrow will have trouble of it's own and yesterday is gone. Concentrate on today. What you CAN do today. What you HAVE TO do today.

It is also important to talk to other people during this time, but don't expect them to understand what you are going through. And let them know that, but you can talk about it ~ it's great therapy. Especially talk to your family. They are your greatest support base, along with your church, and your friends. But most of all, talk to God, He's the only one who truly understands you. Psalm 139 in the Bible was a great inspiration to me.

Let people help you, let them do things for you. They don't know what to say, so let them do. This is more difficult for some of us than for others. I wanted to do everything myself. Mostly to prove to myself that I could still do it. But all I did was use up much needed energy. Let people cook for you, clean for you, wash your clothes. It won't be long and you will be able to do all of those things again. I didn't realize how much I actually enjoyed those things that I used to complain about before.

Perseverance is something you have to *choose* to do ~ not something that comes naturally to most of us. Some of us are optimistic from the beginning and stay that way, but most of us are not. Re-read this section and stay focused on today, on what you need to do to beat this cancer and stay cancer free. *Persevere.* Get help with this if you need it. It will take all your inner strength to fight this and then stay focused on your new healthy lifestyle. You do not want to go through this again, ever! And it will take perseverance to do it successfully. And remember, *the battle for health begins in your mind.* You *can* do this, others have and so can you!

Planning for . . .

Planning for . . .

There are many plans you have to make. Plans for yourself as well as for your family: schedules to work out; who takes the kids to school; who will take care of all of the things you do on a day to day basis. Plan for rest ~ plan for exercise ~ plan for healthy eating ~ and plan for fun! Planning is key. It is something you have to do.

Planning for your dietary health will start in your pantry. Take inventory of what you have and decide what you need for your **low iodine** diet. You will discover healthy items to replace some of those you will discard. The inventory is your starting point.

The recipe section of this book will be helpful in meal planning for your low iodine diet and you can use them when you are not on the diet by using some modifications. Take your time and keep it simple. You don't have to make all the changes at once. But start somewhere and keep going. As you must do with planning for your exercise, start small, but START! There are recipe books that you can purchase and the THYCA Corporation has recipes on their web site. When looking at a recipe, check or add the things that will enhance or boost your immune system.

Then comes the planning for the screening or the treatment. Two weeks prior to your screening or treatment you must go on the low-iodine diet. Your doctor will give you guidelines, but I have found them incomplete as they do little to strengthen the immune system.

BEFORE YOU MAKE ANY CHANGES IN YOUR DIET, IN YOUR SUPPLEMENTS, OR IN YOUR MEDICATIONS, CHECK WITH YOUR DOCTOR. If you should get a doctor who thinks things like your immune system, your diet and your overall health are not important right now, **GET ANOTHER DOCTOR OR AT LEAST A SECOND OPINION.**

The "Low Iodine" Diet

The "Low Iodine Diet"

The importance of this diet is not stressed enough. And the harm that can be done when not followed strictly enough is beyond description. Your body must be iodine-starved for maximum test results and maximum treatment results.

This low iodine diet is important to all thyroid cancer patients. The point of this diet is to deplete your body of its natural stores of iodine. This makes the radioactive iodine treatment more effective. When the radioactive iodine is given, the thyroid will absorb the iodine because it has been very depleted.

There are cookbooks available from several sources. They are wonderful during the time of following the low iodine diet before a scan or treatment. ***However***, I want to concentrate not just on your becoming iodine-starved, I want you to boost your immune system in the process.

Your doctor will put you on the diet for two weeks prior to your scan or treatment, but what many physicians don't tell you is, you cannot resume a normal diet until the scan or treatment has been completed. This sometimes takes another week, sometimes two. *Therefore, the actual duration of this diet is somewhere between fourteen and twenty-eight days.*

Let's explore the reality of this "diet." We call it the **low-iodine diet** because it is virtually impossible to create a no-iodine diet. But we can do low-iodine. And the lower the better. With this diet there is also the risk of lowering other necessary nutrients in the body. Therefore by the third week you can become more tired and your body may begin to crave certain foods.

Your doctor may have different guidelines for this diet. Please check with him/her about your specific needs and guidelines. This is good to go over while you are asking questions and taking notes.

Foods that contain iodine include, but are not limited to:

<><   Iodized salt and sea salt (Because it is difficult to know which restaurants use them, you should NOT eat out during this time.)

The recommendation is to limit eating out, but why take a chance with something as important as this.

<><   Milk and other dairy products including eggs and cheese. Egg whites are acceptable.

The recommendation here is that food containing small amounts of milk or egg may be used. And non-dairy creamers may be used if they do not contain whey.

<><   Seafood, including fish, shellfish, kelp, and seaweed. This group also includes vitamin and mineral supplements if they contain any of these ingredients.

<><   Foods that contain the additives: carrageen, agar-agar, algin, and alginate.

<><   Cured or corned food such as ham, lox, corned beef, or sauerkraut.

<><   Breads made with iodate dough conditioners *(This is tricky because the dough conditioner is usually not listed on the bread labels)*. My recommendation is that you make your own bread, which is easy enough to do with a bread machine.

<><   Foods and medications containing red food dye. This can include orange or brown as well, since they can have red in them. Of course check with your doctor before discontinuing any red, orange or brown colored *medications.*

Also, check your toiletry labels for red dye. Betadine soaps and some shampoos contain red dye. There is also iodine in some topical antiseptics.

I believe this group should include red meat because most of the red meat you buy has some red dye in it to make it look good. It is not normally harmful, but is not worth the risk right now.

<><   Chocolate. Chocolate or anything with chocolate in it is off limits, due to its dairy content.

<><   Molasses and foods that contain molasses.

<><   Soy products such as soy sauce, soymilk, or tofu and foods made from soy products.

Many margarines and oils as well as many processed foods contain soy. So read your food labels very carefully.

<>< Multivitamins and breakfast or diet drinks may also contain iodine. Check with your doctor regarding your multivitamins.

<>< Soft drinks also contain many of the items listed above but may not be listed on the label or the doctor's "no ~ no" list. Especially avoid the dark colored drinks. They are unhealthy anytime.

<>< Many products containing sodium are not specified on the ingredient list. Often the label only reads "sodium." What does that mean? Only the manufacturer knows for sure. ***Low-iodine doesn't have anything to do with sodium.*** Sodium is OK as long as it is not provided as iodized salt.

The information sheet given you by your doctor has examples of foods you can eat. My concern is that you will not be sufficiently "iodine starved" and at the same time, you will become nutritionally starved.

Since everyone's body reacts differently, I believe it is important to take daily supplements during this time so as not to deplete your body of needed nutrients. Supplements should be specific, not multivitamins because most multivitamins contain food dyes or other ingredients you want to avoid. **To ensure that the supplements are all natural, it is best to buy from a health food store, not from your grocery.** Consider with your doctor taking vitamin C & E, Coenzymes Q-10 and Coenzyme A, garlic (the odorless type), Melatonin, B-Complex, as well as Selenium. Your doctor may recommend other helpful supplements. We will explore this in greater detail later.

By now you are asking, "OK, then what can we eat?" Legitimate question and we will address it! The next pages contain food knowledge that will be helpful to you as we go into our recipes and as we decide to be healthy for the rest of our lives. The recipes near the end of the book will help you to eat healthy, and stay focused on your goal. Remember your immune system needs all the help it can get!

Three weeks of this "diet", **can we do it?**

YES WE CAN! And we can feel good doing it!

Food Knowledge

Food Knowledge

Let's put the knowledge we already have together with more knowledge and add things we can do.

Let's go to your food pantry. We'll start with a list of some things that are "No's" and then go into the "Yea's" since there are more of those. Let me say here that if you have Anaplastic carcinoma, you will have to get aggressive ~ and fast! Otherwise the change should be gradual, take it one step at a time. It is not a good idea to get rid of everything in your pantry and start fresh unless you can afford to do so and your family is behind the change one hundred percent. Mine was not ~ they still wanted hamburgers and macaroni and cheese. So make the changes, but be sensitive to your family's expectations. This is a change for them too.

Because of the low iodine diet I will proceed differently than I otherwise would. For example, I'll repeat some food items we discussed in the earlier section.

Since everyone does not have access to whole organic foods, you may have to do the best you can with what is available at your grocery store. However, many grocery stores are beginning to carry more whole and organic foods.

Supplements cannot take the place of healthy foods in helping you stay healthy. They are just what they are called: "supplements."

Pantry "No's"

In this section I will reiterate some of what you read in the section on the low-iodine diet, however, this section will include extra nutritional information.

<><   Sugar-Refined
<><   Caffeine in Coffee, Tea, and Soda

<><   Artificial Sweeteners
<><   MSG products and processed foods
<><   Red Meat
Organically grown meat is fine after your LID
By this I mean meat from animals that have NOT been enhanced by steroids and/or treated with antibiotics.

LID = Low Iodine Diet

<><   Alcohol
<><   Iodized salt and salt by-products
Non-iodized salt is OK to use sparingly
Sea salt is good after your LID
<><   Milk and dairy products including eggs and cheese
OK after your LID
<><   Seafood and seafood products
OK after your LID
<><   Grocery store bought breads
Watch your labels carefully and be sure they are all natural—your whole food grocery store is the best for these products after your LID
<><   Anything containing red dye
Any food dye is not good for your body at any time.
<><   Anything with the additives Carragen, agar-agar, algin, Alginates
<><   Chocolate and anything with chocolate in it
Chocolate does have some healthy components. Try to get organic if you can. Of course this is after your LID
<><   Molasses and anything containing molasses
This product is very good after your LID
<><   Soy products, such as soy sauce, tofu, soymilk, or any other product that contains soy
Soy is another product that is very healthy when you are not on your LID.
<><   Cured or corned foods such as ham, corned beef, etc.
<><   Anything with whey, a dairy by-product
After your LID, watch the intake of whey and make sure it is all natural or as natural as possible
<><   Enriched foods are out, not just for the diet, but also for always. The food is stripped and then nutrients we need are added back in, thus enriched.

Read your food labels carefully! Read not just the product information, but the **actual ingredients list**.

Pantry "Yea's"

As you research on your own, your list may grow. Food allergies will come into play as you look at the lists below and decide which changes you can make and which you must make.

<>< Oatmeal and Cream of Wheat

<>< Herbal tea (except red)
    Red tea can return after your LID

<>< Rice milk
    After your LID

<>< Almond milk
    After your LID

<>< Non-dairy creamer is acceptable *if it does* **not contain whey**.

<>< Pure maple syrup

<>< Whole wheat flour ~ *unbleached*

<>< Pure cane organic sugar
    Sugar is not good for your immune system at any time ~ try to limit your intake.

<>< Barley flour

<>< Olive Oil

<>< Flaxseed oil

<>< Sesame Oil

<>< Aluminum-free baking powder

<>< Organic rice or regular rice including brown rice

<>< Pasta ~ homemade or purchase whole grain or vegetable

<>< Beans ~ fresh, not from a can

    black beans
    black-eyed peas
    kidney beans
    lentils
    pinto beans

navy beans
split peas

Beans are packed with soluble fiber. And because of the ability of beans to keep blood levels stable, it has been shown to reduce the insulin requirements of diabetics. They are a wonderful source of protein, which is important when you can't eat meat or have trouble digesting meat. Beans also help lower blood pressure and reduce the "bad" cholesterol. Beans also contain properties that inhibit the growth of cancer cells. That is because they produce *protease inhibitors*, which is the basic component of beans. They are effective in blocking the formation of colon and breast cancers, to name a few. Scientists have not concluded what the effect is if you already have the cancer. The research is not yet in on that. They can keep many bowel-related problems from developing and can help cure them over time. Remember these are fresh beans that you cook yourself, not processed beans from a can.

Note: The protein is not complete unless beans or legumes are combined with grains; beans and cornbread or beans and rice, for example.

Also, don't be intimidated by the bag of beans that you may not have been exposed to before. They really are very easy to prepare, and can be prepared in advance and can either be frozen or canned.

<>< **Vegetables** ~ let's **not** limit our consumption or our list.

Artichokes
Asparagus
Beets
Brocoli
Brussel Sprouts
Cabbage
Carrots
Cauliflower
Celery
Corn
Cucumbers

Lettuce ~ romaine
Mushrooms
Okra

*Olives and olive oil

The best thing about olives seems to be the oil. Olive oil has been proven to help reduce the risk of heart disease. You can replace margarine, butter and other oils with olive oils and reap many benefits. The evidence is now strong that olive oil also retards cancer growth. Olive oil seems to strengthen cell membranes and make them more stable and better able to resist the free radicals. Olive oil is rich in vitamin E, one of the best antioxidants available. Vitamin E is an *oleic acid,* which is also found in human milk and aids normal bone growth. Olive oil has also been shown to reduce the wear and tear of the tissues and organs of the body and the brain. Olive oil works wonders for heart related diseases as well, because of the polyunsaturated and monounsaturated fats. I won't go into further benefits for other health related problems. But Olive oil has many, many benefits. *If you have not used it before, introduce it into your diet slowly as it can have a slight laxative effect.*

Potatoes
Pumpkins
Radishes
Spinach
Squashes/Zucchini
Summer squash
Winter squash
Sweet potatoes

Tomatoes

Cooked is better than raw for the tomato ~ cook them when they are ripe ~ they are great! These are good for canning and last for quite some time.

Turnips
Yams
Yucca root

I know there are more vegetables. All are beneficial; I've listed some. Add to the list and enjoy!

<>< Fruits—again lets **not** limit our consumption or our list.

Apples

The following is some information on apples;

They lower bad cholesterol.

They lower blood pressure.
As a juice (fresh) it is highly effective in fighting viruses.
They help stabilize blood sugar.
They suppress the appetite without taking away necessary nutrients.
They prevent constipation and help treat diarrhea.
They actually prevent tooth decay.
They contain properties that scientists believe are vital in stopping cancer.
There are indications that apples may fight certain kinds of cancers and block others.

Apple Cider Vinegar
When you are off of the LID

Apricots

Apricots are rich in beta-carotene and fiber. They seem to be better for you dried than fresh. It has been proven that beta-carotene blocks the formation of many forms of cancer.

Bananas
Blackberries
Blueberries
Cantaloupe
Cantaloupe is filled with beta-carotene, fiber, folate, potassium and vitamins B6 and C.
Cherries
Cranberries
Dates

Figs

The Fig's medicinal value is due to its high levels of fiber, magnesium, potassium, vitamin C and other nutrients. Figs also contain B6, which has been shown to help women with their premenstrual stress. The fig's anti-cancer component is *benzalehyde*. The results of testing done on the fig's anticancer component, named above, have been dramatic. Of fifty-five patients involved in a test, seven went into complete remission, and twenty-nine into partial remission. The type of cancer tested was not listed in my research of this study. Fresh figs can be colored golden yellow all the way to deep purple, they come fresh, dried or in tins with juice.

Note: *If you are buying dried figs; check to see if they have been preserved with things you may be allergic to such as sulfites. Sulfites are often used to preserve dried fruits.*

Grapefruit

Grapes

Grapes have an important mineral called *boron*, which helps ward of osteoporosis. *Boron* is now sold as a dietary supplement in health food stores. Grapes also have vitamins A, B and C. The minerals include calcium, potassium and zinc. Grapes fight tooth decay, and can stop viruses in their tracks, and are rich in other ingredients that researchers believe can ward off cancer. The agents in grapes that appear to be antiviral and antitumor are called *polyphenols* and *tannins*. Grapes have high levels of something-called *caffeic acid*, which has been shown to be a strong anti-cancer agent. And raisins have been associated with the reduced rate of cancer deaths among one group of American Senior Citizens tested.

Honeydew Melon
Kiwi
Lemons
Limes
Mangoes
Nectarines
Oranges
Papayas
Peaches

Pears
Pineapples
Plums
Prunes
Raisins
Raspberries
Strawberries
Tangerines
Watermelon

I know there are more fruits. I've listed some. All are very beneficial. Add to the list and enjoy!

There are other healing foods that you can add to your pantry and to your everyday diet.

<>< Honey ~ *Preferably local and* unfiltered.

Honey has many properties. I've learned that archaeologists have discovered an ancient scroll that lists hundreds of remedies for illnesses and injuries. 500 out of the 900 treatments included honey. Honey calms frayed nerves and has been used to help get a good nights sleep as well as bring down a fever when mixed with certain herbs. Honey can kill bacteria and disinfect wounds and sores. Science has also discovered that honey helps asthma sufferers. Honey helps to make us feel better and stimulates the part of the brain responsible for learning. (Honey is not safe for small children)

<>< Nuts

Almonds, Walnuts and Pistachios are the top three, but all nuts have something called *polyphenols, which* researchers have found to help tackle cancer before it begins to spread throughout the body. Other nuts also have this property. Nuts also contain *protease inhibitors,* which researchers say appears to be among the most natural cancer blockers yet discovered. Make sure your nuts are not processed, coated or salted.

Peanuts
Brazil nuts
Cashews
Acorns
Chestnuts
Hazelnuts

Herbs & Spices

Herbs & Spices

Herbal therapies and remedies are probably the oldest form of treatment in the world. They are used to strengthen the body's ability to eliminate cancer cells along with diet, exercise and vitamin and mineral supplements. So lets look at what would be helpful in your **herbal pantry.** The Food and Drug Administration have not evaluated most of these statements. There are however, many studies being done on some of these products as of this writing.

Herbs for General Wellness

<>< *American Ginseng*
Is a generic tonic

<>< *Astragalus*
Also a generic tonic that is said to boost energy.

<>< *Bilberry*
Improves circulation, repairs veins

<>< *Chinese Ginseng*
Generic tonic, energy

<>< *Garlic*
Helps prevent cancer, lowers cholesterol

<>< *Ginkgo Biloba*
Antioxidant, improves circulation and memory

<>< *Gotu Kola*
Improves circulation, healing and memory

<>< *Green Tea*
Antioxidant and tonic, helps prevent cancer

There are many herbal teas that will benefit you greatly. You can mix and match them and try as many as you like. Again, stay away from the red teas until after your low iodine diet.

There is a special tea that I want to bring to your attention, called ESSIAC. It is safe and natural. It is used as a supplement and also concentrates on your immune system. It is rich in vitamins and minerals, which help nourish and strengthen individual cells and molecules. It has no adverse side effects. This is an important tea for your health and well-being. The resource section of this book includes information on how to get this specific tea. *Some health food stores are beginning to carry this product.*

<>< *Milk Thistle*
Repairs liver cells, liver tonic
<>< *Reishi*
Adaptogen, tonic, immune system stimulant
<>< *Siberian Ginseng*
Adaotigen, tonic, boosts energy
<>< *Turmeric (this is also a spice)*
Antioxidant

Herbs Related to the Prevention of
____Other Diseases and Conditions____

<>< *Bilberry*
Prevents hardening of the arteries, hemorrhoids, and poor night vision
<>< *Cranberry*
Great for urinary tract infections
<>< *Evening Primrose Oil*
Essential fatty acid
<>< *Feverfew*
Migraines
<>< *Garlic*
Hardening of the arteries, high cholesterol, high blood pressure
<>< *Ginkgo Biloba*
Memory loss, tinnitus
<>< *Hawthorn*
Angina, congestive heart failure
<>< *Licorice*

Ulcers
<>< *Milk Thistle*
Liver problems
<>< *Saw Palmetto*
Prostate problems
<>< *St. John's-wort*
Mild depression

Not all of these herbs will be in your pantry or medicine cabinet. Check with your doctor and your nutritionist, should you choose to have one, to see if any of these would be helpful for you, particularly if you have other conditions that are not related to your specific thyroid cancer. *Do Not* do this on your own! You and your doctor and/or nutritionist will have to sort through what is best for you, your conditions, your cancer, your treatment and your overall well being.

Now lets get practical and get down to what is in your food pantry that you can use daily or occasionally to enhance the taste of your foods and enhance your immune system.

More Herbs and Spices

<>< Sea Salt *(only use when you are able to use salt again)*
<>< Allspice
<>< Barley

Studies show that barley is one of the three balanced starches (rice and potatoes being the other two), which are rich in complex carbohydrates that fuel the body with energy. Barley also contains *protease inhibitors*. These inhibitors go after cancer causing agents in our bodies and help head them off before cancer can begin to form. There is much research being done in this area. Barley has many other great health benefits and can be used as a substitute for wheat in most recipes.

<>< Basil

Laboratory studies suggest that compounds in basil may help disrupt the dangerous chain of events that can lead to the development of cancers.

<>< Bay Leaves

<>< Cayenne

Cayenne contains *alkaloid capsaicin*, which relieves pain by blocking the chemicals that send pain messages to the brain. It is a spicy powder and when added to food perks up appetite, improves digestion, and relieves gas, nausea, and indigestion. The herb also thins phlegm and eases its passage from the lungs.

Cayenne is also found in tea form if you prefer it that way.

<>< Chili Powder

<>< Cinnamon

Cinnamon contains a chemical called *cinnamaldehyde* that has many benefits one of which is a tranquilizing effect that helps reduce anxiety and stress. It is a very important spice for stress relief.

<>< Cloves
<>< Coriander
<>< Cumin
<>< Curry
<>< Dill Weed
<>< Fennel

<>< Garlic/Garlic Powder

Garlic's medicinal uses have been documented for centuries. It has been linked to the cure and treatment of many diseases and ailments: arteriosclerosis, arthritis, asthma, athlete's foot, baldness, bronchitis, cancer, chicken pox, cholera, the common cold, all the way to malaria, measles and meningitis, just to name a few. Animal tests indicate that fresh garlic might be an effective weapon against a form of breast cancer. Garlic is also very heart friendly and can bring down blood pressure. Another finding in tests revealed that garlic was probably a better antioxidant than vitamin E. The positive effects of garlic are too many to mention here, but this is one heck of a good herb. To reduce the smell, use parsley, to get the garlic off your hands, "wash" them with lemon juice and salt.

<>< Ginger

As an herb, it is the best for motion sickness and nausea, settling the stomach, relieving vomiting, and easing pain. It is wonderful in helping to alleviate the after-effects of chemotherapy as well as external beam radiation.

<>< Hyssop
<>< Maple Syrup *(pure)*

<>< Mint

<>< Mustard *(dry)*

<>< Nutmeg

<>< Onions/Onion Powder/Leek

Like it's cousin, the garlic, it is also noted as a cure-all. Scientists are studying the properties in onions as possible cancer fighters. They already know that *sulfur*, one of the many components in onions seems to work exceptionally well at stopping the sudden changes in cells that often lead to cancer. At the Harvard School of Dental Medicine a project concluded that onion extract stopped the spread of oral cancer cells or destroyed them entirely in animal tests. In a similar study the researcher said that the onion extract might prevent at least some forms of cancer from ever starting in the first place.

<>< Oregano

<>< Paprika

<>< Parsley

<>< Rosemary

<>< Sage

<>< Tarragon

<>< Thyme

<>< Turmeric

Turmeric is packed with antioxidants, including vitamins A, C, and E, which we know have far-reaching benefits.

<>< Wheat

Wheat bran is loaded with crucial B vitamins and protein. Wheat germ is rich in fiber, B vitamins, iron, magnesium and zinc. Also included are chromium, manganese and vitamin E. Wheat guards us against colon cancer. The benefit of this cancer-fighting tool is that wheat bran creates bulkier stools, which then move through the colon faster, picking up unwanted chemicals as they go. That tremendously improves the chances of avoiding cancer.

I have only touched on the benefits of some of these herbs and spices. There are of course more and there are benefits to all of them. Attempting to list them would take us too far from our main topic. Nevertheless, I wanted to give you some insight to the benefits. Most can be used on the low iodine diet without a problem and there is no limit on how much of the beneficial foods you can eat.

Supplements

Supplements

In some cases, supplementation with a nutrient is a simple and less expensive alternative to obtaining it solely through food. Supplementation can cause trouble for someone who decides that if some is good, more is better. Talking supplements sensibly, with your doctor and/or nutritionists supervision for safety is the key to reaping their benefits. You, your doctor and/or nutritionist will have to decide what, if any supplements you should be taking at this time.

<><   Coenzyme Q10

There is a book by Ray Sahelian, MD titled *Coenzyme Q10* that goes into the many benefits of this enzyme. Benefits that range from the heart to the thyroid. Researchers at the Department of Internal Medicine, Fujita Health University School of Medicine, in Aichi, Japan did a study about coenzyme Q10 and vitamin E in relation to thyroid cancer. The researchers wrote, "These findings imply that vitamin E and coenzyme Q10 as antioxidants play some roll in thyroid follicular cell function." Your doctor should determine the dosage of the enzyme; especially if you have other conditions and more so if you are going to have chemotherapy.

<><   Coenzyme A
<><   Colostrum
<><   Dimethylglycine
<><   Garlic
<><   Inositol Hexophosphate
<><   Melatonin
<><   Proteolytic Enzymes
<><   Selenium

<>< Shark Cartilage
<>< Vitamin A
<>< Carotène
<>< Vitamin E
<>< Vitamin C
<>< Calcium
<>< Vitamin D

<>< Acidophilus

Acidophilus is the primary friendly bacteria found in the intestinal tract and vagina. It is responsible for producing *acetic acids* that lower the natural pH in the intestines, which, in turn discourages the growth of other bacteria. The bacteria, along with other beneficial bacteria, produce an antibiotic-like substance that works against viruses, protozoa and fungi. They work to protect the body from invaders. It is found in supplement form or in yogurt that contains live and active cultures. It has been called "nature's antibiotic" and has many benefits and uses. Entire books have been written on this bacteria, so you can do a little more research and your doctor may be able to give you more information.

<>< Flaxseed Oil

According to the Word Health Organization, Omega-3 fatty acids from vegetable sources such as flax oil are essential for good health. We've heard much about these Omega-3 acids in recent years and more and more benefits are being found. If you become deficient in these acids many things can go wrong with the body from acne to arthritis to mental illness and even obesity and vision disorders, just to name a few. There are about 50 known disorders that are associated with the lack of this fatty acid in the body. The deficiency in children is being linked to ADHD and behavioral problems. There has been extensive research done on it in recent years.

<>< Multienzyme Complex
<>< Vitamin B Complex

There is one more thing I want to go into here that has to do with supplements and their overall health benefits.

Glyconutrients. Research on these glyconutrients began in the 1960's. Since then the study has grown as technology has developed. The science of the glycoprotien synthesis can be explored in great detail. There is a web site I will reference for your information. Basically these glyconutrients are special patent-pending product that protects healthy cells and aids in cell communication. Protecting healthy cells is something we all want to know more about. I could write a book on these nutrients alone. However, many scientists and researchers have already done this. Please check into this as a supplement. Your doctor may also research this product at the referenced web site. This has been a great aid to my well being and will be helpful to you and your doctor. I provided information on this product to all of my doctors right away, because I saw the difference in my health right away.

Juicing Does Help

Juicing Does Help

Juicing at one time was a hot commodity. Juicers were flying off of the shelves and everybody was doing it. Now it seems less desirable because it takes time and effort. But the time and effort are well worth it, especially when you are trying to get your immune system back on track and get all of the cancer toxins as well as the treatment toxins out of your system.

No group of people has a greater need for the benefits of fresh fruit and vegetable juice than those with cancer. Chemotherapy and radiation expose healthy cells as well as cancer cells to free-radical damage. The result is depletion of valuable antioxidant enzymes and nutrients.

Fresh juice contains a wide range of substances referred to as *anutrients*. These are enzymes, pigments like carotene, chlorophyll, and flavanoids, and accessory food components. The anutrients are responsible for many known as well as unknown benefits of food.

More and more experts are realizing that it's not just the "essential nutrients" that are important, but that anutrients may possess the greater effect in protecting against cancer.

The American Cancer Society's key dietary recommendations to reduce the risks of cancer include vegetables such as cabbage, broccoli, Brussels sprouts, and cauliflower.

The study of food is an open field. Each year more and more anutrients are being discovered showing that they produce remarkable health benefits. Most of the anutrients in fruits and vegetables have yet to be discovered.

Juicing not only provides important antioxidant nutrients that can protect against the damage of radiation and chemotherapy it also provides a wide range of anutrients. Juicing is used as part of the nutritional support program for the cancer patient in many cancer treatment centers across the country.

If you don't have a Juicer, the best place to buy one is at a health food store. Make sure that the Juicer is stainless steel and does not have any aluminum parts. Also, low powered Juicers cannot juice some of the harder vegetables such as carrots. A salesperson in your health food store will have knowledge of the product and can help you select what you need at a price you can afford. A good book on juicing is also helpful and will have some beneficial recipes for you to enjoy. It is a good investment in your health. The juicer can be used by itself or in conjunction with a blender. Some fruits such as bananas don't have a lot of juice and therefore are not recommended for your juicer. Adding the juice from your juicer with bananas in a blender would be the best option.

Organic produce is the best for juicing, just as it is the best for eating, however not all of us can get the organic produce. Do the best you can with what you have and can get. Some grocery stores are now carrying more organic items. When you don't have the organic, you can run the risk of juicing and ingesting the pesticides that are in and on the fruits and vegetables. There is a wash available in most stores to remove most of these pesticides from your fruits and vegetables. My suggestion is that you use it. It is very helpful in removing topical toxins as well as the wax that is sometimes put on fruit to keep it looking fresh while it is being stored for long periods of time. So if you can't buy organic, use the wash to clean up your produce. You can use this wash on organic fruits and vegetables as well if you so desire.

Don't mix your fruits and vegetables. The only exception to this is the apple. For some reason it is palatable with vegetables as well as with other fruits.

This is not just for juicing it is for your meals as well. When you are having fruit don't have vegetables, and when you are having vegetables don't have fruit at the same meal. This is helpful in digestion and the metabolizing of nutrients.

In the next section of this book are the recipes that will help you through your "low-iodine" diet and boost your immune system. You can review the food knowledge again if you have questions concerning the recipes and the choice of ingredients that will be included. Feel free to experiment on your own and come up with things that you and your family like. You and your body will benefit from all the things we went over. Your whole body is sick, so lets get your whole body well.

The Bible states in 3 John 1:2 (NIV)

"Beloved, I pray that in all respects you may prosper and be in good health, just as your soul prospers."

There are many options available for cancer treatment and there are no guarantees. My hope is that this book will benefit you and that you will search out the options that are right for you. No one therapy is right for everyone. Search out what conventional medicine has as well as alternative treatments and create your own program. No one should pressure you into a specific treatment. You should only feel pressured to educate yourself to what is available for you. I hope this book has been a stepping-stone in that process. This book is not exhaustive ~ it is intended to stimulate you to gain more knowledge.

As I complete this book I have been cancer free for three years. I'd like to tell you that I'm in great shape, but truth be told, I am still working hard at being healthy and staying on track with all the things I spoke about in this book. My whole body was sick and it is taking some time to get my whole body well. I have other conditions that hinder me as well. And of course I didn't know then what I know now, so my recovery is taking longer, but my expectations are high. I want to feel better than I did before I had cancer, and I should. The fact is that **I am cancer free right now**! And that is exciting news.

I pray you will persevere and be healthy. I believe that lifelong health is a goal we can all attain.

If I have just one last bit of advice it's don't give up! Join the support groups. Exercise with friends. Enjoy your family and friends. And keep what goes into your body as healthy as possible. My best wishes go out to all of you out there who are facing some sort of thyroid condition or battling thyroid cancer of some kind.

May God be with you all!

Recipes

Fruit Smoothie—Before and after your
"Low Iodine Diet" unless you customize it.

Anytime Pancakes
Apple Cinnamon Cream of Wheat
Apple/Carrot Juice
Black Beans & Rice
Black-Eyed Pea Salad
Broiled Oven Potatoes
Chicken Rollups by Joe
Chicken and Dumplings by Granny
Cinnamon Baby Carrots
Cinnamon Toast
Creamed Spinach by Grandma
Creamy ~ Dreamy Cauliflower
Fruit Crisp
Fruit & Oats
Fun Fruit Salad
Italian Style Green Beans
Lemon Chicken
Mashed Sweet Potatoes
Noodles
Oven Fried Chicken
Oven Roasted Potatoes
Penne With Broccoli & Garlic
Pineapple Chicken
Salad & Dressings

Sautéed Vegetable Medley
Spinach & Apple Salad
Steamed Veggie Combo
Sweet Potato Casserole
Veggie Supreme Salad

Recipe Notes

Breadcrumbs can be made in a food processor. You can flavor them with parsley, oregano and garlic powder. Your local bakery may also have fresh breadcrumbs. Make sure you enquire about content.

Keep on hand some low-iodine snacks, such as:

Fresh Fruit

Carrot Sticks ~ washed and cut ~ ready to eat

Raisins

Matzo crackers ~ unsalted ~ can be found in the Kosher aisle of your grocery store

Unsalted Nuts ~ look for these in the baking aisle or at your health food store

Homemade breads and muffins (made ahead of time by you to assure they are low-iodine)

Try to make up batches of allowed snacks and freeze in portion sizes for yourself. There are times when you won't want to eat a meal, or you are just too tired. Eating an allowed snack food is better than going off of the diet.

When eggs are called for in a recipe ~ use the whites only and double them.
2 egg whites for 1 egg.

Fruit Smoothie

½-1	frozen banana (quartered)
1	cup frozen strawberries, blueberries (or other desired fruit)
2 TBS	Natureade Vegetable Protein Powder
2 TSP	Kyo/Barlean's Green Powder
1-2 TBS	Barlean's Flaxseed Oil
20-40	drops of ConcenTrace Mineral Drops
¼ TSP	Ambrotose powder**
½ TSP	probiotic (Natren or Kyodophilus)

1-cup   ice, **optional**

2 cups   juice (fresh if possible) or rice, soy, or almond milk, or 1
cup or water and 1 cup of juice/milk

Directions:

Combine ingredients in order listed above and blend until completely blended (approximately 1½ minutes). Amounts of fruit, juice, milk or water and ice can be varied to give desired consistency.

**Most of the ingredients can be found at your local health food store. The exception is the Ambrotose Powder. That ingredient is available at the online address below.

www.mannapages.com/AWolfe

***This shake as is can only be used when you are *NOT* on the "low iodine" diet as some of these materials contain iodine with the exception of the Ambrotose Powder, the Flaxseed oil and of course the fresh fruits. You can alter the ingredients to fit what you need at this time for your benefit and go to this version after your LID.

This Smoothie was developed by Lifestyle for Health and can be found on their web site.

Anytime Pancakes

Have these pancakes for breakfast with fruit, for lunch with veggies, or for dinner
with whatever you are hungry for.
As a snack they are my favorite

4   cups of flour
4   egg whites
3 to 3 ½ cups of water
Olive Oil

Wisk together making a very thin dough.
Heat enough olive oil to cover the bottom of a frying pan.
Pour batter into hot oil and allow to fry.
Flip and fry the other side.
Place on paper towel to soak up the oil.

Eat hot or cold. With cinnamon and sugar, jelly, fruit, vegetables or plain.

Apple Cinnamon Cream of Wheat

One Serving

1 Granny Smith Apple or an apple of your choice.
Cut into small pieces into a cereal bowl.
Sprinkle with approx. 3 TBSP of wheat germ.
(optional)
Then sprinkle with ¼ TSP sugar and ½ TSP cinnamon and stir.
(sugar is also optional)

Cook Cream of Wheat according to directions with water.
Add 1 TSP of sugar and ½ TSP cinnamon after cooking.
Pour over the apple mixture in the cereal bowl and ENJOY!

Apple/Carrot Juice

This recipe is of course for those of you who have a juicer available. If you have a friend who has one, try theirs and see how much you like it!

4 Carrots
2 Apples (Granny Smith)
Cut into wedges.
Put through the juicer as directed by the manufacturer.

Alternate carrots and apples to get a well blended juice.

To this mix you can add:

¼ inch slice of ginger and/or
¼ tsp cinnamon or other vegetables such as: spinach radishes beets

Have fun experimenting!

Black Beans & Rice

2 cups of Black Beans—uncooked
6 cups of filtered or purified water
2 bay leaves ~ whole
4 cloves of garlic crushed
1 TBSP oregano
2 TBSP lemon juice ~ freshly squeezed

Combine Black Beans ~ water ~ bay leaves into a large pot. Bring to a boil.
Reduce heat and cover.
Simmer for approximately 2 hours (stirring occasionally to keep beans from sticking).
After the 2 hours ~ add herbs and spices (except lemon juice) and cook for 5
    minutes.
Using a potato masher, mash about ¼ of the beans to give them a thicker texture.
Add lemon juice and cook for another ½ hour.
Serve over organic rice with some hot bread! Yummy!

Black-Eyed Pea Salad

1   cup cooked fresh black-eyed peas.
Rinse w/ filtered water & drain.
1 ½ cups chopped, peeled tomatoes
1   cup fresh slightly cooked corn
¼   cup thinly sliced green onion or leek
1/3   cup olive oil
2   TBSP balsamic vinegar
3   TBSP fresh squeezed lemon juice
4   TBSP snipped fresh thyme or 1 TSP dried
¼   TSP pepper
1   TBSP snipped fresh Rosemary or 1 TSP dried

In a large mixing bowl ~ stir together black-eyed peas, tomatoes, corn, green onion and cover. Chill for 24 hours.

Dressing: Combine olive oil, lemon juice, vinegar, thyme, rosemary and pepper ~ shake well. Chill for 4 to 24 hours. Just before serving pour dressing over salad mixture. Toss gently and enjoy!

Broiled Oven Potatoes

9   potatoes (all purpose or red potatoes)
Olive Oil
1   garlic clove ~ crushed
½   TSP onion powder
pepper to taste
1   TBSP dried basil
½   TSP dried oregano
½   TSP dried parsley

Wash potatoes thoroughly and slice.
Place sliced potatoes into a casserole dish coated with olive oil.
Add spices and mix ~ adding olive oil as needed for an even mixture.

Broil until brown on top.

Chicken Rollups by Joe

1 small spanish onion ~ chopped large carrots ~ sliced ¼ inch thick
2 TBSP olive oil
Sauté together until tender
1 LB Chicken filets ~ cut into strips
Onion powder ~ garlic powder ~ lemon pepper (to taste)
Cook in non-aluminum cookware until chicken is cooked through and is tender.

½ cup shredded lettuce ~ romaine
1 chopped tomato
1 chopped avocado (optional)

Wrap all of the above in a flour tortilla and savor the flavor.

After your LID ~ add some cheese or dressing or anything else you wish.

Chicken & Dumplings by Granny
(Revised Edition)

1 Whole chicken (skinned)
Enough water to cover the chicken in a very large pot.
A pinch of non-iodized salt and pepper to taste
Place chicken and water into a Very Large pot and cook until the chicken comes off of the
     bone easily.
Remove chicken from pot.
De-bone chicken and return to the pot.
To chicken and broth ~ add:
4   carrots ~ sliced or chunked
2   celery Stalks ~ chopped
1   onion ~ finely chopped
¼   cup fresh parsley ~ chopped
2   bay Leaves
2   cloves garlic—minced
1   TSP Turmeric
½   TSP Cayenne
1   TBSP Olive Oil

Cook until carrots are tender.
While this is cooking make the dumplings.

Dumplings

2 Cup flour
2 Egg Whites
1 Cup Water
A pinch of non-iodized salt (optional)
Extra Flour to keep dough from being too sticky.

Mix dough and roll dough out on a floured board to ¼ inch thickness (dough will be
    slightly sticky)
Cut into strips and place into boiling broth.
Cook for approximately 10 to 15 minutes.

Cinnamon Baby Carrots

1 Bag of baby carrots
1 tsp cinnamon
1 ½ cups of water

Combine ingredients in a saucepan.
Cover and simmer until carrots are at desired tenderness.

This is a great side dish for anything ~ anytime.

Cinnamon Toast

Your own bread ~ sliced fairly thin.
Sprinkle with cinnamon and sugar.
Rub cinnamon and sugar into the bread just a little.
Toast in a toaster oven. If you are making a large quantity broil in regular oven.

The sugar gives it a nice crunchy texture!

This is great to compliment your breakfast or just anytime as a snack to satisfy a
    craving.

Creamed Spinach by Grandma (Revised)

1   bag of fresh (organic if possible) spinach
¼   cup onion ~ finely chopped
1/8 cup olive oil
¼   cup flour
½   TSP paprika
¼   TSP pepper
1   TSP garlic powder
(or one fresh clove of garlic ~ pressed)
½ to ¾ cup of spinach fluid (drained from cooking)

In a saucepan cook spinach in approximately 1 cup of water. Cook spinach until
    spinach is soft and tears easily.
Drain into a bowl to keep the fluid.
In the saucepan, combine olive oil and onions, cook under low heat until onions
    start to sweat.
Add the flour and stir with a whisk to make a creamy paste.
Add the juice from the drained spinach ~ just enough to make a creamy sauce ~
    using the whisk to assure creamy texture.
Add the spices.
Finally add the spinach and stir until well blended. Add juices or water as needed.
Simmer over medium low heat for 15 to 20 minutes with cover on the saucepan.
Stir occasionally to keep from sticking.
Add small amounts of water as necessary.

(This can be frozen and used later)

Creamy ~ Dreamy Cauliflower

1 head of cauliflower (organic if possible)
Cook in large saucepan in filtered water until tender.
(Drain cauliflower ~ saving the fluid)

4 TBSP of acceptable margarine substitute
Melt in saucepan

Add 1/3 cup of flour (may add up to 3 TBSP as needed) stirring constantly.

(In place of the margarine substitute and flour, you can use some of the cooked cauliflower and mash enough to make the sauce creamy.)

Add juice from the cauliflower and some Chicken stock to desired thickness using a whisk to keep the mixture creamy.

Salt (non iodine) and pepper to taste.
Add a dash of parsley ~ fresh or dried

Bring to a boil and add the cauliflower.

Let sit for about an hour or so and heat just before serving.

(This can be frozen and used later)

Serve this over the "Anytime Pancakes" for a delicious "Anytime Meal."

Fruit Crisp

5 cups of sliced and peeled: apples ~ pears ~ peaches ~ apricots
** *blueberries ~ cherries*
2 to 4 TBSP sugar
½ cup regular rolled oats
½ cup packed brown sugar
¼ cup flour
¼ TSP ground nutmeg/ginger/or cinammon
¼ cup margarine (salt free)
¼ cup freshly shelled nuts ~ chopped
¼ cup wheat germ (optional)

Oven to 375°
Place fruit into an 8 x 8 baking dish and stir in the sugar.

Topping: In a medium sized mixing bowl combine: Oats
Brown Sugar
Flour
Spice

Cut in margarine until mixture resembles coarse crumbs. Stir in nuts and sprinkle over fruit filling.

Bake for 30 to 35 minutes or until the fruit is tender and the topping is golden brown.

**For *Blueberry or Cherry* Crisp: Place fruit in an 8 x 8 baking dish and stir in 3 tbsp of sugar and 3 tbsp of flour. Mix the blueberries, sugar, and flour. Then continue with the recipe above.

Fruit & Oats

¾ cup fresh quick rolled oats or oatmeal
1 apple, pear, peach, or other fruit

Cut fruit into bowl with oats.

Add 2 TBSP wheat germ (optional)

Add 1 TBS pure cane sugar
Add 1 TBS cinnamon (optional)

Mix well!

Add boiling water to desired consistency.

Great for breakfast or lunch!

After your LID use Rice or Almond Milk for a variety of tastes and flavors.

Fun Fruit Salad

Combine your favorite fruits. As many or as few as you desire.
Slice or chunk as desired.
Add some nuts and/or wheat germ for an added crunch.
Add the juice of one fresh lemon and stir.

Allow the salad to sit for about an hour or so to allow the fruits to expel some juice.

Stir again just before serving
Serve with a slice of fresh bread or muffin.

After your LID ~ you can serve with sour cream.

Italian Style Green Beans
(Revised edition of Laurie Perrault's recipe)

1 lb Fresh Green Beans ~ snapped and cut
2 TBSP olive oil
2 cloves garlic ~ cut up small
½ cup of fresh bread crumbs
(to bread crumbs add garlic powder, dried basil and dried oregano)

Cook and drain green beans ~ saving the juice.
Place olive oil and garlic in a deep fry pan ~ and simmer until garlic is sweating.
Add green beans and simmer about 5 minutes.
(Add juice from green beans to keep from sticking)
Add breadcrumbs and simmer for another 5 minutes.

Lemon Chicken

3 lemons
2 TBSP olive oil
½ cup of Fig Spread (check ingredients) ~ optional
¼ cup white wine ~ optional
¼ cup water
2 whole chicken breasts (skinned)
2 TBSP chopped fresh parsley or 1 TBSP dried
black pepper to taste
salt (non iodine) to taste
allspice to taste

Preheat oven to 400 degrees.

Squeeze juice from one lemon into a bowl.
Add olive oil, fig spread, white wine and water.
Stir with whisk.
Thinly slice the other two lemons and place in a small casserole dish or baking
    pan.
Place chicken pieces on top of lemon slices.
Pour the lemon mixture on top of chicken and lemon slices.
Then sprinkle spices on top of chicken.
Bake for 45 to 55 minutes until chicken is done through.
Serve with rice or noodles.

Mashed Sweet Potatoes

Up to 5 sweet potatoes ~ boiled and peeled
¼   TSP cinnamon
1/8 TSP nutmeg any or all   } any or all
1/8 TSP ginger
1   TBSP brown sugar
½   TSP fresh lemon juice
¼ to ½ cup fresh orange juice

Add ingredients to boiled and peeled potatoes and mash together until smooth
    and creamy.

Serve in place of regular mashed potatoes with any dish.

Noodles

1 cups of flour
2 cup water
3 egg whites
An additional little bit of water

Mix ingredients ~ dough will be tough!

Rinse the pasta press in cold water before pressing the dough through ~ makes
    for a smoother press.

Press dough into boiling water—boil approximately 20 minutes.

As an alternative ~ if you don't have a pasta press.

Roll dough out to 1/16 inch or so on a floured board.
Cut dough into small thin strips.
Carefully place strips into boiling water and add and additional 5 minutes or so
    to cooking time.

Oven Fried Chicken

1 boneless chicken breast ~ skinned
1 medium onion ~ diced small
1 garlic clove ~ pressed
1 cup breadcrumbs mixed with:
¼ TSP basil
¼ TSP oregano
¼ TSP cayenne
¼ TSP paprika
¼ TSP pepper
*salt to taste ~ non iodized
egg whites

Olive Oil

Whisk egg whites until frothy.
Add onion and garlic to egg whites and whisk again.

Dredge chicken breasts in egg mixture.
Then roll chicken in breadcrumb mixture.

Place in a well oiled (olive oil) covered casserole dish.

Bake for 30 minutes in a 350-degree oven.
Uncover and bake another 15 to 20 minutes for crispy chicken.

Can use Corn Flakes instead of breadcrumbs after your LID for a crispier crust.
Do not cover chicken when using Corn Flakes.

Oven Roasted Potatoes

1   lb medium sized red potatoes
¼   cup olive oil
4   TBSP fresh squeezed lemon juice
1   TSP dry oregano or 1 TBSP fresh oregano ~ minced
5   TBSP thin lemon zest (not the outer peel ~ the white peel)
½ TSP garlic powder
¼ TSP pepper
¼ TSP turmeric

Wash potatoes thoroughly using filtered water or vegetable wash.
Quarter unpeeled potatoes and place in a large bowl.
In a small bowl, blend the rest of the ingredients.
Pour contents of small bowl over potatoes and stir until potatoes are well coated.
Pour potatoes in a large baking dish in a single layer.
Roast in a 375-degree oven for 40 minutes shaking the pan at 20 minutes to
    relocate the potatoes.

Penne With Broccoli & Garlic

1 lb broccoli flowerets
1 ½ cups olive oil
16 garlic cloves ~ minced
½ TSP red pepper flakes (optional)
1 lb penne or any short pasta ~ cooked and drained.

Blanch broccoli in boiling water for 7 minutes.
Drain, rinse with cold filtered water and drain again.
Chop into small chunks.
Heat oil in a large skillet.
Add broccoli, garlic, red pepper flakes and cook over medium low heat for 10 to
    15 minutes.

Toss with HOT pasta and serve immediately!
What a treat for your taste buds!

Pineapple Chicken

½ cup fresh pineapple juice (use juicer)
1 cup filtered water
4 chicken filets
½ to 1 cup fresh pineapple chunks
1 TSP allspice

Rub each piece of chicken with ¼ TSP of allspice.
Put pineapple juice and water into a large skillet.
Put chicken into pineapple/water mixture.
Cook thoroughly.
Place pineapple chunks into pan when chicken is done and heat.
Add water as necessary due to evaporation.

You can add flour or corn starch to make a sauce to serve over rice, pasta or
   potatoes.

After your LID you can add molasses for a tasty treat.

Salad and Dressings

*There is nothing like a nice garden salad made with fresh greens and fresh
   vegetables.*
*Mix as many as you like using fresh romaine lettuce and spinach leaves as a
   possible base.*

Nutty Dressing

½ cup chopped nuts
Remember that buying nuts for baking usually alleviates the salt issue
½ cup extra virgin olive oil
¼ cup distilled vinegar or balsamic vinegar
¼ cup fresh squeezed orange juice

Place all ingredients into a blender.
Process until smooth.
Pour over hot or cold vegetables or salads.

Vinaigrette Plus Dressing

1/3 cup olive oil

¼ cup honey

2 TSP Balsamic vinegar

1 TBSP Flaxseed Oil

1 ½ TSP fresh squeezed lemon juice

2 garlic cloves ~ minced

small pinch of sugar

pepper to taste

Combine ingredients in a jar with a tight-fitting lid and shake well. Pour over salad just before serving.

Spinach & Apple Salad

2 cups of fresh torn spinach

2 cups of fresh torn romaine lettuce

¼ cup sweet onions

1 apple—sliced with peel still on

raisins (optional)

Combine ingredients and top with Nutty Dressing.

Variation

2 cups fresh torn spinach leaves	Mix	olive oil, 1 fresh garlic clove ~ crushed,
1 ~ 3 apples ~ sliced		and 1 TBSP flaxseed oil
Fresh walnuts		Mix Well
1 spanish onion ~ sliced	Pour	over salad and serve immediately.

Sautéed Vegetable Medley

2 TBSP olive oil
2 large carrots
1 small zucchini
1 small summer squash
1 small onion
½ red pepper
1 celery stalk
1 tomato
1 small apple
½ spanish onion
A few mushrooms
A few spinach leaves

1   clove garlic
¼ TSP pepper
¼ TSP turmeric
¼ TSP cayenne
1   TBSP dried parsley

To olive oil add the sliced vegetables and apple.
Sauté until vegetables are tender.
Add spices and garlic, heat through and serve.

Serve over something or have it by itself.
A great slice of bread always goes well with this meal.

This is an immune system booster.

Steamed Veggie Combo

1 sweet potato
2 large carrots
1 zucchini
1 squash some broccoli flowerets some cauliflower flowerets

Cut all of the above into chunks.

Place in a steamer basket.

Then, to the water add a clove of garlic, rosemary, and thyme.

Steam until vegetables are at desired tenderness.

To water add some pepper and flour. Stir with whisk to make a smooth sauce.
Serve sauce over the vegetables.
This can also be served by adding vegetables to the sauce and then served over
    rice.

Sweet Potato Casserole

3   sweet potatoes ~ boiled and peeled (organic if possible)
2   oz of olive oil
¼   TSP cinnamon
1/8 TSP nutmeg
1/8 TSP ginger
3   TBSP brown sugar
½   fresh pineapple ~ cut small or crushed
½   TSP fresh lemon juice
1   egg white

Mix all ingredients together well.
Put ingredients in a well oiled (with olive oil) 2 quart casserole dish.
Bake in a 350-degree oven for 30 minutes.
Remove from oven and add large marshmallows to top and return to oven until
    marshmallows brown on top ~ 5 to 10 minutes.

Veggie Extreme Salad

1 bag of vegetable spiral noodles
Cook according to directions.
Cool noodles with filtered cold water

Add the following ingredients:
½ cup coarsely chopped cauliflower flowerets
½ cup coarsely chopped broccoli flowerets
2 medium grated carrots
1 sprig of fresh parsley ~ finely chopped
¼ cup fresh spinach leaves ~ finely chopped
1 large plum tomato ~ sliced and cubed
1 large yellow squash ~ sliced and cubed

Dressing:

4 TBSP olive oil
2 TBSP distilled or balsamic vinegar
¼ TSP dill
¼ TSP basil
1/8 TSP tarragon
1/8 TSP sage
1/8 TSP thyme
1/8 TSP mint

Dried
or
Finely
chopped
fresh

Mix in a glass shaker ~ mix well.
Pour over salad and let set for one hour before serve

I hope you enjoy all of the recipes and that they give you a nice variety over the duration of your "Low Iodine Diet" and beyond. Remember that you can experiment with all of the knowledge you have now.
God be with all of you!

Recommended Reading

and Researching

Books:

Townsley, Cheryl. *Food Smart, Eat Your Way To Better Health*. Denver, Lifestyle for Health, 1997.

Townsley, Cheryl. *Cleansing Made Simple*. Littleton, CO: Lifestyle for Health, 1998.

(Cheryl Townsley's books and tapes are available from Lifestyle for Health, 1-303-794-4477.)

Balch, Phyllis A, and Balch, James F. *Prescription for Nutritional Healing, Third Edition,* 2000.

Blaylock, Russell L, M.D. *Health and Nutrition Secrets that can save your life*, 2002.

H. Jack Baskin, M.D. *How Your Thyroid Works*. Adams Press, Chicago IL. 1991

Michael Garcia, M.D., Donald A Meier, M.D., and Charles I. Taylor, M.D. *Your Thyroid Gland—A Guide for Thyroid Patients*. Associated Endocrinologists, P.C. 1993

Tapes:

Dr. Lorraine Day, an internationally acclaimed orthopedic trauma surgeon and best selling author was for 15 years on the faculty of the University of California, San Francisco, School of Medicine as Associate Professor and **Vice Chairman of the Department of Orthopedics.** She was also **Chief of Orthopedic Surgery** at San Francisco General Hospital and is recognized worldwide as and AIDS expert. She has been invited to lecture extensively throughout the U.S and the world and has appeared on numerous radio and television shows including **60 Minutes, Nightline**, CNN Crossfire, **Oprah Winfrey, Larry King Live, The 700 Club**, Art Bell Radio Show, USA Radio Network, Three Angels Broadcasting Network and Trinity Broadcasting Network.

Her Tapes Include:

"Cancer Doesn't Scare Me Anymore!"

(As a physician who developed cancer herself, Dr. Lorraine Day was well aware that physicians are more afraid of cancer than patients are, because doctors KNOW that chemotherapy, radiation and surgery are NOT the answer to cancer. She will help you understand, all the confusing medical jargon you will hear from the doctors. By following the orderly system of evaluation that she presents, you can then make calm, intelligent decisions about the best treatment methods for you.)

Double Blind, What Science Can't See
You Can't Improve On God!
Diseases Don't Just Happen!
Drugs NEVER Cure Disease
Believing is Seeing!

You can reach Dr. Day at *www.drday.com,* or through:
    Rockford Press,
    PO Box 8
    Thousand Palms, CA 92276.
    (800) 574-2437.

Organizations:

AACE
1000 Riverside Ave.
Suite 205
Jacksonville, Florida 32204
(904) 353-7878

American Foundation of Thyroid Patients
18534 North Lyford

Katy, Texas 77449
(281) 855-6608

American Thyroid Association
Townhouse Office Park
55 Old Nyack Turnpike
Suite 611
Nanuet, New York 10954
(914) 623-1800

The Endocrine Society
4350 East West Highway
Suite 500
Bethesda, Maryland 20814
(301) 941-0200

Thyroid Foundation of America, Inc.
Ruth Sleeper Hall, RSL 350
40 Parkman Street
Boston, Massachusetts 02114-2698
(800) 832-8321

The Thyroid Society for Education and Research
7515 South Main Street
Suite 545
Houston, Texas 77030
(800) 849-7643

Thyca: Thyroid Cancer Survivors' Association, Inc.
P.O. Box 1545
New York, NY 10159-1545
(877) 588-7904

Thyca's services include an ever-growing roster of local support groups, an informative web site (listed below), several e-mail discussion groups for thyroid cancer survivors and family members, a one-on-one peer support program, publications (including a low iodine cookbook), and much more. All of these services are free and available to everyone. Funding comes from membership dues, as well as from grants and contributions from businesses and individuals. Thyca also sponsors an annual conference for thyroid cancer survivors, family members, and friends. The Thyca web site has details.

Websites:

www.glycoscience.com,
This site is maintained as a public service to provide educational information on dietary supplements and the science behind them, specifically glyconutrients. These were only touched on in this book, but I recommend that you and your doctor visit this website.

Should you be interested in ordering any products containing these nutrients please visit my website at: *www.mannapages.com/Awolfe.*

www.thyca.org,
They offer Person-to-Person Support, Local Support Groups, E-Mail Support Groups, Publications, an Award-Winning Web Site and Conferences. No matter what type of thyroid cancer you have, they are there to offer support, education, and encouragement to you and your family. Contact them:
ThyCa: Thyroid Cancer Survivors' Association, Inc.
PO Box 1545
New York, NY 10159-1545
Call Toll Free: 1-877-588-7904
Visit: *www.thyca.org*
E-Mail: *thyca@thyca.org*

www.lifestyleforhealth.com,
Contact Dr. Cheryl Townsley, N.D. at:
      LifeStyle for Health
      6520 S. Broadway
      Littleton, Colorado 80121

      Call: 1-303-794-4477
      Fax: 1-303-794-1449
      E-Mail: *info@lifestyleforhealth.com*

LifeStyle For Health offer a variety of services such as; Personal Health Coaching, Urine Panel Assessment, Dental Materials Testing, Body Scan, Hair Scan, "Body By Design" Facilitator Training, Foot Reflexology, Chair Massage, Exercise Classes, and many Educational Materials, as well as a Health News Flash that you can have sent directly to your E-Mail address. Dr. Cheryl Townsley is a widely published author and has appeared on numerous television and radio shows.

www.Thyrogen.thera.com
   This site offers more information on the Thyrogen option in your thyroid testing.

www.bilsuebest@aol.com
This site offers information on the Essiac Herbal Tea
Bill & Sue Best are also Essiac Distributors.
      Best Enterprises
      41 Plain Street
      Rockland, MA 02370
      781-871-9844

Essiac Tea information can also be found at:
      Rene M. Caisse Research Institute Canada
      P.O. Box 23155
      Ottawa, Ont. Canada K2A 4E2

Manufacturer Information:
Essiac International
164 Richmond Road
Ottawa, Ontario K1Z 6W2

Phone: (613) 729-9111

Information on the 714X I mentioned can be obtained through:
CERBE Distribution Inc.
5720, Mills
Rock Forest
Quebec, Canada J1N 3B6

Phone: (819) 464-2883 or 564-0492
Fax: (819) 564-4668
E-Mail: *cerbe@cerbe.com*
Internet: www.cerbe.com

Resources

American Association of Clinical Endocrinologists. *The Thyroid Nodule. Hypothyroidism. Hashimoto's Thyroiditis. Thyroid Carcinoma. Radioiodine Therapy*. Prepared by the AACE.

American Thyroid Association. *Cancer of the Thyroid*. 1996

Bernard Ward. *Healing Foods from the Bible*. Boca Raton, Florida 2001

Cathryn Conroy. *The Toughest Part of Exercising Is . . .* CompuServe News

Cheryl Townsley. *Food Smart, Eat Your Way To Better Health*. Denver, Lifestyle for Health, 1997.

Cheryl Townsley. *Cleansing made simple*. LFH Publishing, Littleton, CO, 1997.

Cheryl Townsley. *Food Puzzle*. LFH Publishing, Littleton, CO. 2001

Deanne Tenney. *Nature's Antibiotic, Acidophilus*. Pleasant Grove, UT 1996

Endocrine Disorders & Endocrine Surgery. *Thyroid Nodules. Thyroid Goiter, Enlargement of the thyroid. How Your Thyroid Works. Your Thyroid. Thyroiditis, Inflammation of the Thyroid Gland. Your Parathyroid. Thyroid Function Tests, Normal Laboratory Values. Thyroid Nodule Ultrasound. Common Tests to Examine Thyroid Gland Function*. 1997. <http:// www.EndocrineWeb.com

Genzyme Corporation and Knoll Pharmaceutical Company. *Thyrogen Support Kit*. 1999

GlycoScience & Nutrition. *Glyconutritionals : Implications for Cancer*. Coppell, Texas 2000

Jones Pharma Incorporated. *Hyperthyroidism.*

Knoll Pharmaceutical Company. *The Thyroid Gland and Your Health*. 1997

Linda B. White, M.D., Steven Foster, and the staff of Herbs for Health. *The Herbal Drugstore*. Rodale 2000

Lisa Richwine. *Drug That Sends Radiation to Tumors Up for Review*. 2001

Michael T. Murray, N.D. The Complete Book of Juicing. Rocklin, CA 1992

National Cancer Institute. *Eating Hints for Cancer Patients*. NIH Publication 1994

Need a Second Opinion? *Patient Information*. RG Images. 1996

Patricia Hausman, and Judith Benn Hurley. *The Healing Foods*. Pennsylvania: Rodale Press, Emmaus 1989.

Phyllis A. Balch, CNC., and James F. Balch, M.D. *Prescription for Nutritional Healing, Third Edition*. New York: Avery 2000

Ray Sahelian, M.D., and Jack Challem. All about coenzyme Q10. New York: Avery 1998

Rene M Caisse, R.N. *The Story of Essiac by Rene M Caisse R.N.; Her Healing Journey; 1888-1978*. Resperin Corporation. 1997

RENEW LIFE Digestive Care Newsletter. *Digestive Care and Cleansing*. Tarpon Springs, Florida

Richard A. Passwater, PhD, and Jack Challem. All about antioxidants. New York: Avery 1998

Russell L. Blaylock, M.D. *Health and Nutrition Secrets that can save your life*. Albuquerque, NM 2002

Suzanne Cliché. *714X*. 2001

ThyCa.org. *How is Thyroid Cancer Treated? Treatment Option Overview. What is Thyroid Cancer? Word Index*.

University of Massachusetts. *Iodine Precautions*. Patient Information

*Winning the Battle Within * Glyconutrients: The missing link to optimal health*; Video for Educational Purposes Only; Available through Mannatech Inc.; Produced by WinkStar, Inc. Hoffman Estates, IL